T0211090

Police Services

Paresh Wankhade • David Weir
Editors

Police Services

Leadership and Management Perspectives

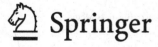 Springer

Editors
Prof. Paresh Wankhade
Edge Hill Business School
Edge Hill University
Ormskirk
United Kingdom

Prof. David Weir
Edge Hill Business School
Edge Hill University
Ormskirk
United Kingdom

ISBN 978-3-319-37777-3   ISBN 978-3-319-16568-4 (eBook)
DOI 10.1007/978-3-319-16568-4

Springer Cham Heidelberg New York Dordrecht London
© Springer International Publishing Switzerland 2015
Softcover reprint of the hardcover 1st edition 2015
This work is subject to copyright. All rights are reserved by the Publisher, whether the whole or part of the material is concerned, specifically the rights of translation, reprinting, reuse of illustrations, recitation, broadcasting, reproduction on microfilms or in any other physical way, and transmission or information storage and retrieval, electronic adaptation, computer software, or by similar or dissimilar methodology now known or hereafter developed.
The use of general descriptive names, registered names, trademarks, service marks, etc. in this publication does not imply, even in the absence of a specific statement, that such names are exempt from the relevant protective laws and regulations and therefore free for general use.
The publisher, the authors and the editors are safe to assume that the advice and information in this book are believed to be true and accurate at the date of publication. Neither the publisher nor the authors or the editors give a warranty, express or implied, with respect to the material contained herein or for any errors or omissions that may have been made.

Printed on acid-free paper

Springer International Publishing Switzerland is part of Springer Science+Business Media (www.springer.com)

Acknowledgements

There are a number of people to whom we would like to express our sincere gratitude for this ambitious project. Firstly, we would like to thank our authors who are well regarded for the expertise in their fields. They range from senior academics, chief constables, serving and ex-police officers & police staff, and independent practitioners. To bring them all together is a key highlight of this volume, and to this end this is a book by the people who lead and manage the police services and their opinions are important in informing the policy and guiding the practice. Secondly, to the team at Springer Publishing, in particular, we are grateful to Janice Stern and Christina Tuballes. Thirdly, to Prof. George Talbot and Prof. James O'Kane at Edge Hill University for supporting the project. Lastly, to our families for allowing us at different periods, to develop this book.

Paresh Wankhade, Lancashire, UK
David Weir, Lancashire, UK

Contents

Contributors

Andrea Bishop Kent, UK

Ginger Charles Institute for Spirituality and Policing, Modesto, California, USA

Modesto Junior College, Modesto, California, USA

Julian Constable Anglia Ruskin University, Cambridge, UK

Andrew C. Fisher Liverpool Hope University, Liverpool, UK

John G. D. Grieve Portsmouth University, Portsmouth, UK

Barry Loveday University of Portsmouth, Portsmouth, UK

Jacques de Maillard CESDIP and Institut Universitaire de France, University of Versailles-Saint-Quentin, Versailles, France

Timothy Meaklim University of Ulster, Coleraine, United Kingdom

Rowland Moore Merseyside, UK

Jon Murphy CC Merseyside Police, Merseyside, UK

Peter Neyroud Jerry Centre for Experimental Criminology, Institute of Criminology, Cambridge University, Cambridge, UK

John M. Phillips Liverpool Hope University, Liverpool, UK

John W. Raine Institute of Local Government Studies, University of Birmingham, Birmingham, UK

Susan Ritchie MutualGain, Essex, UK

Colin Rogers International Centre for Policing and Security, University of South Wales, South Wales, UK

Jonathan Smith Devon and Cornwall Police, Devon, UK

Paresh Wankhade Edge Hill University, Ormskirk, UK

David Weir Edge Hill University, Ormskirk, UK

About the Editors

Paresh Wankhade is the Professor of Leadership and Management at Edge Hill University Business School. He is a founding editor of International Journal of Emergency Services and is recognised as an expert in the field of emergency management. His research and publications focus on analyses of strategic leadership, organisational culture, organisational change and interoperability within the public services with a special focus on emergency services. His publications have contributed to inform debates around interoperability of public services and challenges faced by individual organisations.

David Weir is Visiting Professor at Edgehill University, and has held Chairs at several universities including Glasgow, Bradford, Liverpool Hope, UCS and SKEMA in France. He has worked with several police forces and has published extensively on risk management and undertook a major study with the Police Federation on the work of police sergeants in the UK. He has supervised more than sixty PhD theses on aspects of management and has written several books and many journal articles.

Part I
Context and Background

Chapter 1
Introduction: Understanding the Management of Police Services

Paresh Wankhade and David Weir

Introduction and Background

This book is the first of a three volume series on the management of the three blue light emergency services (Police, Ambulance and the Fire & Rescue Services) being published by Springer, USA. This volume aims to provide a broader management understanding of the police services which would be of equal interest to a wide audience including students, academics, practitioners, professionals including the leadership & management practitioners in police forces without compromising the rigour and scholarship of the content. We have invited experts in their particular fields to address the chosen themes, both in the theory and practice of the functioning of the police services in the UK and abroad. The key thinking in this volume is to provide a broad understanding of the major management issues relevant to police services in the UK along with an international perspective. Admittedly it is a difficult endeavour to cover all the possible management themes in a single volume such as this but we are confident that the chosen topics will provide an expert view and a rounded understanding and insights into the management of police services.

More attention is being paid now to the management research on police services given the policy and practice implications of the challenges and changing context of policing. Several factors have contributed toward the need for a better understanding of the role and contribution of the police services in the wider criminological settings. The pressures on police budgets and the resulting implications for service delivery have been well rehearsed. The deteriorating global security climate and the growing numbers of cyber-crime cases coupled with lower public confidence

P. Wankhade (✉) · D. Weir
Edge Hill University, Ormskirk, UK
e-mail: Paresh.Wankhade@edgehill.ac.uk

D. Weir
e-mail: weir53@gmail.com

© Springer International Publishing Switzerland 2015
P. Wankhade, D. Weir (eds.), *Police Services*, DOI 10.1007/978-3-319-16568-4_1

and low staff morale is likely to add more pressures on the use of the police services. The Mid Staffordshire Hospital Inquiry (Francis 2013) and the Keogh Review
(NHS England 2013) both highlighted a cultural transformation of the hospital and
emergency/urgent care services in England. This calls for a similar understanding of
the police services thus making this project particularly timely. The chosen themes
in this volume will help to outline the social, cultural, and political context in which
the police services is to be understood. This volume covers issues of theory, policy
and practice and raises questions, some of which are intrinsically controversial.
Each of the chapters seeks to engage with the current debates about the direction of
travel. The contributors also examine the latest development in their chosen field
of enquiry. This volume thus aims to set out the management understanding of the
police services as a significant sub-discipline of emergency management and also
provide a basis of learning and teaching in this field.

Changing Context of Policing

In the UK, we are currently witnessing two contradictory trends: that of decline in
the policing and crime statistics in the UK amidst escalation of global violence, and
the growing threats to world security climate. The international peace is threatened
by a range of events, sometimes not connected but each posing a significant policing
challenge and having implication for an appropriate police response. For instance,
the turmoil from the continuing civil war in Syria, the latest round of escalation of
violence in the Arab-Israel conflict including the deteriorating situation in Iraq and
the rise of a new militant group are a few cases to note. Another totally unconnected
danger is from the pandemic threat of the new deadly *Ebola Virus* from West Africa,
posing a significant challenge to policing with global ramifications.

In the UK, the latest Crime Survey in England and Wales (CSEW) for the year
ending March 2014 revealed that there were an estimated 7.3 million incidents of
crime against households and resident adults (aged 16 and over) for the year ending March 2014 (see Fig. 1.1). This represents a 14% decrease compared with the
previous year's survey and is the lowest estimate since the CSEW began in 1981
(Office for National Statistics ONS 2014). However, this is in contrast with the police recorded crime figures which show no overall change from the previous year,
with 3.7 million offences recorded in the year ending March 2014. Prior to this
police recorded crime figures have shown year on year reductions since 2002/2003
(ONS 2014).

There is no consensus among experts about the reasons for fall in the crime figures and a range of factors including the decline in binge drinking, rising alcohol
prices and the state of the economy have been reported (Travis 2014). Jon Boutcher,
the national policing spokesman on surveillance was reported (Dry 2014) to argue that drop in crime figures was misleading since lot of criminal behaviour has
moved online, where much of it goes either unreported or undetected and warned
of being complacent to the dangers of cyber-crime. Furthermore, the CSEW (previ-

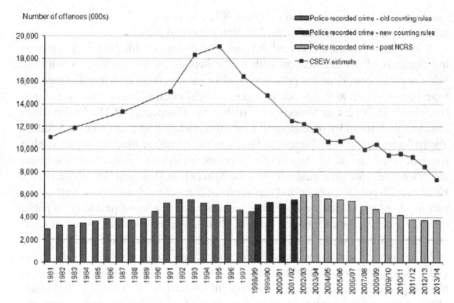

Fig. 1.1 Police recorded crime, 1981 to 2013/14. (Source: Office for National Statistics-Crime in England and Wales, Year Ending March 2014)

ously British Crime Survey) in use since 1982 has undergone changes from being a research tool to be seen as a system of performance management (Hough et al. 2007). Significant methodological limitations of using surveys as research tools in measuring the performance of public services have been reported (Cantor and Lynch 2000). Recently, Feilzer (2009) examined whether the data collected through the BCS (now CSEW) can be considered as valid and reliable indicators of local police performance. Her analysis showed that perceptual measures included in the BCS and used as performance measures are 'under-conceptualised, invalid, context dependent, strongly related to social-demographics and are unreliable'.

Meaningful performance reporting by police forces and in wider public services has been under considerable scrutiny (Shane 2010; Wankhade and Barton 2012; Loveday 2008; De Bruijn 2002; Wankhade 2011; Andrews and Wankhade 2014) with the MORI 2007 survey (IPOS MORI 2008) reporting how a large proportion of public do not believe crime is falling and more than 60 % of the public have not heard of the Police Inspection Agency (Her Majesty's Inspectorate of Constabulary). The Casey Report (2008) describes that less than 1 % of respondents relied on published statistics as their primary source of information to find out whether the crime in their region was increasing or decreasing. Information about policing is increasingly available outside police agencies through different sources including national TV and newspapers, official websites, and social networking sites (O'Connor 2010). Research on factors that drive public confidence conducted by the College of Policing (formerly National Policing Improvement Agency) and Metropolitan

Police (NPIA/Home Office Final Report 2010; Neyroud 2010) further highlighted the significance of good quality information put out to public.

It has been generally accepted that opening dialogue with public and improving channels of communication with public acts as another form of contact and helps improve confidence in policing (Bradford et al. 2009). A string of allegations have been levelled at the police in recent months eroding public trust in policing (Hillsborough 2012; Her Majesty's Constabulary of Inspection 2011). British media has been dominated by several stories including ranging from undercover Scotland Yard officers trying to influence the family of the murdered black teenager Stephen Lawrence in London, to the arrest of a police officer for lying about witnessing the "Plebgate" row involving MP Andrew Mitchell in Downing Street; the alleged Hillsborough police cover up and the arrests of current and former police officers as part of the Met's Operation Elveden investigation into alleged payments to public officials in return for information (Maybin 2014). The 'reassurance' aspect of policing offers another perspective in improving public confidence (Skogan 2009).

Police services are also witnessing a new challenge on the institution of the Police Federation of England and Wales which is a staff association for all police constables, sergeants and inspectors. An Independent Review led by Sir David Normington (2014) has provided a series of recommendations (pp. 65–68) to improve trust and accountability, foster openness and transparency and improving financial priority with a detailed timetable to re-write the terms and reference of the federation's constitution. Furthermore, acting on a whistle-blower's case from the Metropolitan Police Service, the House of Commons Public Administration Select Committee (PASC) published a damning report about the massaging of the Police Recorded Crime statistics (PASC 2014). The report recommended to the UK Statistics Agency (UKSA) acting in response to the evidence exposed by PASC's inquiry, to strip Police Recorded Crime statistics of the quality designation 'National Statistics' (PASC 2014, p. 52).

Historically, concerns over police accountability and the control of wide ranging police discretion impacting on individual's civil liberties are as old as policing itself (Feilzer 2009; Gaines and Cains 1981; van Maanen 1973). A 'tripartite' structure of police accountability which distributed responsibilities between the Home Office, the local police authorities and the chief constable of the force was in vogue till recently. In November 2012, 41 Police and Crime Commissioners (PCCs) were publicly elected across England and Wales, something billed as the most significant constitutional reform in the last five decades. The PCCs became responsible for a combined police force area budget of £ 8 billion to hold Chief Constables and the force to account; effectively making the police answerable to the communities they serve (Association of Police and Crime Commissioners 2014). The real impact of the elected PCCs on accountability relationships is still being debated (Keasey and Raine 2012; Sampson 2012; Joyce 2011) with Lister (2013) arguing that the new 'quadripartite' governance framework for police institutional accountability may generate pressures on PCCs to interfere in what Chief Constables do.

Important lessons are to be learned by the police services from the Frances report (NHS England 2013) into the patient deaths at the Mid Staffordshire NHS Foundation Trust which re-emphasised the need for organisations to create and maintain the right culture (Foster 2003) to deliver high-quality care that is responsive to users' needs and preferences. Loftus (2010) argued that the underlying world view of officers displays remarkable continuity with older patterns, and police culture endures because the basic pressures associated with the police role have not been removed questioning the increasingly accepted view that orthodox conceptions of police culture no longer make any sense. Many of these changes will require a different style of policing, one which "fosters the trust and confidence of local communities and meets their concerns and expectations" (Karn 2013, p. 5). Understanding police culture(s) nevertheless offers important insights into the nature of the organisation and how it deals with issues of legitimacy, accountability and future direction of travel (Waddington 1999; Barton 2003; O'Neil et al. 2007; Cockcroft 2013).

Against the changing landscape of policing, the role and function of the police is also changing. The police mission has become broader and more complex, embracing functions more commonly associated with other agencies (Karn 2013). Yet the public (and political) expectation from police services still centres on crime protection. This volume provides a timely discussion of some of the key management issues being confronted by the police services.

Aims and Plan of this Book

This volume provides a mature understanding of an important public service. Thus, one of the aims of this volume is to invite a new generation of management scholars to explore the study of the police services. This volume will also appeal to a range of students (both undergraduate and postgraduate) studying organisational theory as well as social sciences, sociology, economics and politics, community engagement, emergency planning and disaster management. The book offers critical insights into the theory and practise of strategic and operational management of police services and the related professional and policy aspects. For a large number of staff working in the emergency care settings, the growing calls for professionalisation of the service (through closer links with HEIs) and the recognition to reflect on their own personal development, this volume seeks to provide an authoritative source on the management of the police services addressing the knowledge gaps. This volume will equally appeal to a growing audience of independent practitioners and consultants, both in the UK and working around the world.

One of the other aims of this volume is to bring together, top-quality scholarship using experts- academics, practitioners and professionals in the field, to each of the chosen topics. Admittedly this was an ambitious task and we have been really fortunate to have an assembly of authors who are well regarded for the expertise in their fields. They range from senior academics, chief constables, serving and ex-police officers & police staff, and independent practitioners. To bring them all together is a key highlight of this volume and to this end this is a book by the people who lead and manage the police services and their opinions is important in informing the policy and guiding the practice. The contributors have written from different perspectives of critical academics to chief executives and policy experts and there is much to be gained from reading chapters in 'conjunction with each other, contrasting different perspectives and approaches' (Newburn 2003, p. 7). We are immensely grateful to them for their untiring work that has gone to produce this volume and feel confident that it will do justice to the complexities of the chosen themes. All the chapters have been completed in 2014 and hence draw upon the latest evidence and research base available on the chosen topic. The chapters are based in the practical experiences of the authors and are written in a way that is accessible and suitable for a range of audiences.

In dealing with these issues, the volume is divided into four parts. Part 1 provides the context and background to this volume. Chapter 1 examines the context of policing and states the aims of this volume. In Chap. 2, John G.D. Grieve explores the historical perspectives in policing. His chapter looks back to the founding fathers of policing in the eighteenth and nineteenth centuries and considers whether their thinking has any application in the governance reforms of the early twenty-first Century. He provides a practitioner's reflective view of where policing came from and what is the significance for governance, leadership and management now of those earliest days? He argues in his piece that Robert Peel deserves much of the credit for the practical development of the emerging framework, even if not the precise labelling of them as Peel's *Nine Principles of Policing* that he has sometimes been given. But he should be given the credit as an artificer building on what had been begun earlier rather than as a completely original thinker as Douglas Hurd's work advises us (Hurd 2007). Reith's articulation remains helpful as an ideal. These Principles, he concludes, have relevance and find resonance even today.

Part 2 of this volume deals with the 'doing' of the police services in preventing crime and providing order in the society. Five key themes are examined. In Chap. 3, police leadership is examined by Andrew Fisher and john Phillips. They argue that the police service is facing a crisis of public confidence amidst a range of current challenges. The service is being faced, not only, with political and fiscal challenges, but also cultural & structural problems, and societal issues have threatened the principles of policing by consent and legitimacy. They contend that the crisis can be seen to be the result of failed leadership and policing strategies over decades, and the danger is that there will be more of the same. Case for a new model of policing that recognises the value of engaging communities to re-build confidence and assist in the single mission of reducing crime, based on 'trust, norms and networks' is made in their piece. This chapter examines the challenges and explores what needs to be done to make this happen.

In Chap. 4, Julian Constable and Jonathan Smith examine the contentious theme of police occupational culture. The study of police occupational culture has revealed a wealth of hitherto unknown and unseen aspects of the working life of police officers. In the social science literature this culture is often linked to many of the problems that have been evident in the police organisations of England and Wales. In this way, the authors argue, initial training environment is often considered a place where otherwise 'good' new recruits are inducted into a sub-culture that is pernicious to themselves, the service and those they police. The case study of initial training described in their piece, indicates a complex picture where examples of practice and behaviour that is both progressive and problematic are found. Some specific recommendations are made with regard to changes that might be considered for future iterations of initial police training by the force in question and the service as a whole.

In Chap. 5, the issue of community engagement is investigated by Susan Ritchie. She argues that adopting a deficit model of public service delivery where services 'fix' communities rather than build on the strengths they have, is just not working. She provides a personal practitioner perspective of the future of democracy in the UK with a particular focus in the way public services understand the communities they serve. Going beyond public confidence and satisfaction ratings more democratic initiatives such as Citizens' Charters, pledges and local area agreements offer greater opportunity to reconnect the state with the individual and to re-think the feminist phrase of 'the personal is political' so that it can be applied to all public services. She concludes that by developing new skills to listen differently to the communities they serve, police services can act as the 'enablers' of active citizenship to reduce demand and improve social capital.

In Chap. 6, we include two practitioner contributions on the important themes of Managing Diversity in the police and that of Risk Management. Rowland Moore first explores the issue of equality and diversity in police forces in a short piece. He argues that being immersed in a culture dominated by people who might be different by gender, sexuality, race or disability, presents significant additional personal challenges. Some are obvious from the outset and are by definition easier to deal with whereas others are more insidious involving practices seemingly ingrained in organisational culture. He contends that in the final analysis, policing appears to be heavily populated by values underpinned in conservatism—a political philosophy or attitude emphasizing respect for traditional institutions, distrust of government activism and opposition to sudden change in the established order. In the second piece, Andrea Bishop examines the 'frontline' view of the management of risk in policing. For her, strong leadership and operational credibility are crucial components for senior managers to readily possess and to successfully deliver against in policing. She argues that confidence and trust of the public is an absolute priority and is at the heart of British policing. Members of the public will always turn to the police in times of need and it is in these difficult times that we must ensure that we get it right. She concludes that a proactive approach to listening coupled with strong leadership can help to make sensible decision about addressing risks and managing them.

Part 3 of the volume explores current debates in policing through four key themes. In Chap. 7, Jon Murphy explores the essence of policing from his perspective of a Chief Constable in the North West of England. He argues that the police service has always been excellent at training its people; investing huge amounts of money and resources on how to do 'stuff', about the law, codes of practice, about process and the tactical delivery. But whilst they train well, they are not so good at teaching people to think about policing, about its mission and its legitimacy. From him, there is nothing revolutionary or clever about the basic philosophy of policing, but quite the opposite-"I don't believe in fixing what is isn't broken and I don't believe in change for change sake." Notwithstanding various challenges, not least of shrinking budgets, he concludes that police forces maintain and build on their reputation by keeping the public safe, and by being openly accountable for their actions.

The issue of police accountability is examined by John W Raine in Chap. 8. The election across England and Wales in November 2012 of 41 Police and Crime Commissioners (PCCs)—one for each police force area outside London marked the launch of an intriguingly novel approach to police governance at the local level. The new arrangements have replaced the tradition of committee-style model, originally of council-led 'police committees', and subsequently (from 1964) of separate 'police authorities' (comprising a mix of nominated councillors and other local appointees). The new PCCs are directly-elected individual office-holders whose role it is to provide the strategic leadership and democratic governance for police and crime-related activity, including the key role of holding the chief constable and the local police force to account on behalf of the public. Drawing from empirical analysis of interviews with a sample of PCCs, the various accountability relationships are evaluated. It is concluded that each of the PCCs was also driven by desire to acquire good personal understanding of public expectations about policing and crime reduction and to ensure that such understandings could be reflected in their own prioritisations of policing resources and in their approach to the role more generally.

Our next author Barry Loveday deals with the subject of police modernisation in Chap. 9. His key argument is that the future police management in an age of austerity should be ready to experiment with innovative developments that provide a level of service expected of it by the public. The modernisation debate cannot be about police establishment any longer but should concentrate on both police deployment and more effective resource allocation. He argues that if the evidence suggests that further reductions in police establishment, when balanced by increases in non-sworn civilian staff undertaking more operational roles could increase police effectiveness, then this should be addressed. It is further contended that in an environment that now increasingly recognises the significance and impact of anti-social behaviour on both individuals and communities, there is a clear case for further evaluation of alternatives to a police response to it. The chapter suggests some possible avenues which could provide the basis for both an effective collaboration between police and local authorities while also providing a more effective response to community demands and victim's needs.

The subject matter of 'personal resilience and policing is next examined in Chap. 10 by our experts Jonathan Smith and Ginger Charles. Police services around the world face many kinds of challenges which often impact directly, and not always positively, on the people who work within these organisation. These are often manifested through increasing levels of stress, burnout and PTSD (Post traumatic stress disorder). In this chapter the authors have explored how resilience may be useful in assisting people to not only cope with these challenges but thrive and prosper in this environment of uncertainty and rapid and constant challenge and change. The chapter develops further, the idea of holistic resilience, and explores the component parts to this, using a holistic framework called the Global Fitness Framework. It investigates some of the benefits to developing greater resilience at individual, organisational and societal level and concludes with an exploration of how the different elements to resilience might be developed by police organisations.

Part 4 of this volume presents perspectives on the future of the police services, both in the UK and internationally. Rather than long chapters, these contributions are intended to be shorter pieces to capture greater variety and expertise surrounding the future of policing. In the context of UK, three perspectives are discussed in Chap. 11. The first contribution by David Weir and Paresh Wankhade provides a counter-view on the arguments put forth by some of our contributors on the future of policing. They also comment about the nature of police work and the changing societal context for policing. The piece contends that some of these debates do not all point necessarily in the same direction and many contentious themes still resonate and are not resolved notwithstanding an emerging consensus among police officers and experts. They raise the issues of legitimacy, resourcing and technology and argue that the ultimate objective for everyone should be a society in which citizens feel safe and criminals feel anxious. They conclude that the responsibility for that ultimately lies with both police and the public they serve.

In the second piece, Tim Meaklim argues that in complex times policing still holds a central role in the maintenance of law and order. There is an uncertain future for policing especially as the organisational concept; practice and function of the police are undergoing transition. His piece explores the current complex socio-political, technical and operational environment of policing, before considering possible key topics that will impact upon the future of policing including terrorism, cyber-crime, organised crime and threats created by climate change or infectious diseases. Finally it considers how leaders and the police organisation can forecast, plan, and manage the future policing response to meet the changing environment, whilst remaining flexible and able to work through uncertainty.

Our third expert opinion is provided by Peter Neyroud who draws attention to a deep crisis in public policing which has been precipitated by the combination of fiscal austerity, falling crimes and changing crime patterns. He argues that the crisis is affecting the legitimacy of the institution and requires a new approach from police leaders. To him, the new approach centres around the police taking ownership of the science of policing and building new professional practice based around evidence and supported by a reformed police education. For this to happen, he contends, that the police officers and police leaders will need to value science as a key determinant of their choice of tactics and strategy and a vital part of the qualification framework for any applicant to or practitioner in policing. For police leaders confronting the challenges of the "perfect storm", it is essential task for police to own, deploy and develop the science of policing.

In Chap. 12, we present two contributions addressing international perspectives for police services. Our first author, Colin Rogers argues that policing is not a stand-alone activity, but is affected by many different global changes and other social factors. Consequently police leaders now and in the future will need to be aware of potential global activities in order to provide an adequate response to changing circumstances. Further, police organisations will need to be flexible and adapt to these changes in order to remain effective. This chapter considers the potential changes and their impact that will provide future challenges for police leaders. Our second expert Jacques de Maillard, exploring the French National Police, argues that at all levels of police management, the use of dashboards and performance indicators is usual, both internally to manage personal and vis-à-vis external partners. His text aims to question the effects of the uses of these indicators by taking the example of the French National Police. After having briefly described the modes of operation of police organizations affected by the deployment of these indicators, he analyses the impact on police work and interactions within the police organisation as well externally. The piece especially focuses on the rationalisation process at work, the perverse effects associated to these new policy instruments and the internal controversies associated to them.

Limitations of the Current Project

As editors there were a few difficult decisions we had to take; the biggest one was to decide what to include in the volume and what was to be excluded. We are also conscious about the possible disagreements about the final contents of the volume and what else could or should have been covered. Furthermore, even the scope of some of the chapters could have been more detailed and capable of being examined in a greater detail. The chosen themes do not aim to cover the whole gamut of issues which could be applied to the management of police services. Nonetheless they provide a fair representation of topics that concern us in our scholarly research and teaching. We firmly believe that they represent opportunities for both teaching and practice to reflect on these issues. We also seriously deliberated upon the choice of the authors and their backgrounds. In the end we were convinced that a choice reflecting a balance between academic experts and senior practitioners would bring greater criticality and reflection to the understanding of the chosen themes. Rather than having rigid guidelines over chapter style and structures, we saw greater relevance in a 'light touch', free flowing style of each of the chapters in presenting the contrasting perspectives from academics and practitioners. We are of the opinion that this approach worked better in a work like this though it will be for our readers to judge whether we were correct in our methodology. Similarly we could have paid more attention to the developments in policing outside England though there remains a strong comparative element from Europe.

Future Research Agenda

Police services play a crucial role in maintaining order in the society and in preventing crime. But the context in which they currently operate within the criminal justice system is increasingly becoming fragmented, complex and politically contested. The challenges of funding, training, online-crimes and cultural transformation are now felt globally. The need to learn and adapt from suitable models of police service delivery across the globe have never been greater. We sincerely hope that this volume will trigger greater interest in the understanding of one of the most important of public services. We aim to further work on a comparative element outside the UK and invite interested colleagues and partners to join the quest of the management understanding of a service which is so important to the society.

References

Andrews, R., & Wankhade, P. (2014). Regional variations in emergency service performance: Does social capital matter? *Regional Studies*. doi:10.1080/00343404.2014.891009.

Association of Police and Crime Commissioners. (2014). Role of the PCC. Available at http://apccs.police.uk/role-of-the-pcc/. Accessed 7 Sept. 2014.

Barton, H. (2003). Understanding occupational (sub) culture- a precursor for reform: The case of the police service in England and Wales. *International Journal of Public Sector Management, 16*(5), 346–358.

Bradford, B., Jackson, J., & Stanko, E. (2009). Contact and confidence: Revisiting the impact of public encounters with the police. *Policing & Society, 9*(1), 20–46.

Cantor, D, & Lynch, J. P. (2000). Self-report surveys as measures of crime and criminal victimisation. *Criminal Justice, 4,* 85–138.

Casey, L. (2008). *Engaging communities in fighting crime*, crime and communities review. London: Cabinet Office.

Cockcroft, T. (2013). *Police cultures: Themes and concepts*. Oxon: Routledge.

De Bruijn, H. (2002). *Managing performance in the public sector*. London: Routledge.

Dry, T. (2014). Crime is not falling, it's moved online, says police chief. *The Telegraph*, 22nd April 2014.

Feilzer, M. Y. (2009). Not fit for purpose! The (Ab-) use of the British crime survey as a performance measure for individual police forces. *Policing, 3*(2), 200–211.

Foster, J. (2003). Police cultures. In T, Newburn (Ed.), *Handbook of policing Chapter 9* (pp. 196–227). Cullompton: Willan.

Francis, R. (2013). *Mid staffordshire NHS Foundation trust public inquiry. Final Report*. London: The Stationery Office.

Gaines, L. K., & Cain, T. J. (1981). Controlling the police organization: Contingency management, program planning, implementation and evaluation. *Police Studies: An International Review of Police Development, 16,* 16–26.

Her Majesty's Constabulary of Inspection. (2011). *Without fear or favour: A review of police relationships*. London: HMIC.

Hillsborough Independent Panel. (2012). *Hillsborough the report of the Hillsborough independent panel*. London: HC 581, The Stationery Office.

Hough, M., Maxfield, M., Morris, B., & Simmons, J. (2007). The British crime survey over 25 Years: Progress, problems, and prospects. In M. Hough & M. Maxfield (Eds.), *Surveying crime in the 21st century*. Cullompton: Willan.

Hurd, D. (2007). *Robert Peel*. London: Weidenfeld and Nicolson.

IPOS MORI. (2008). *Closing the gaps crime and public perceptions. Ipsos MORI*. London: Social Research Institute.

Joyce, P. (2011). Police reform: From police authorities to police and crime commissioners. *Safer Communities, 10*(4), 5–13.

Karn, J. (2013). *Policing and crime reduction: The evidence and its implications for practice*. London: Police Effectiveness in a Changing World Project, Police Foundation.

Keasey, P., & Raine, J. W. (2012). From police authorities to police and crime commissioners. *International Journal of Emergency Services, 1*(2), 122–134.

Lister, S. (2013). The new politics of the police: Police and crime commissioners and the 'operational independence' of the police. *Policing, 7*(3), 239–247.

Loftus, B. (2010). Police occupational culture: Classic themes altered times. *Policing and Society, 20*(1), 1–20.

Loveday, B. (2008). Performance management and the decline of leadership within public services in the United Kingdom. *Policing: A Journal of Policy and Practice, 2*(1), 120–130.

Maybin, S. (2014). Do the public still trust the police? *BBC News Magazine,* 25th March 2014.

Newburn, T. (2003). *Handbook of policing.* Cullompton: Willan.

Neyroud, P. (2010). Protecting the frontline: The recessionary dilemma. *Policing, 4*(1), 1–6.

NHS England. (2013). *Transforming urgent and emergency care in England: Urgent and emergency care review,* Phase 1 Report, NHS England: Leeds.

Normington, D. (2014). *Police federation independent review: Final report, The trusted voice for frontline officers, The Royal Society of Arts.* London: RSA.

NPIA/Home Office Final Report. (2010). *The national workforce modernisation programme.* London: The Stationery Office.

O'Connor, D. (2010). Performance from the outside. *Policing, 4*(2), 152–156.

Office for National Statistics. (2014). *Crime in England and Wales, Year Ending March 2014, Statistical Bulletin.* London: ONS.

O'Neill, M. E., Marks, M., & Singh, A. (2007). Police occupational culture: New debates and directions. *Sociology of Crime Law and Deviance,* Vol. 8. Emerald.

Public Administration Select Committee. (2014). *Caught red-handed: Why we can't count on police recorded crime statistics. Thirteenth report of session 2013–14. HC 760.* London: The Stationery Office.

Sampson, F. (2012). Hail to the chief? How far does the introduction of elected police commissioners Herald a US-Style politicization of policing for the UK? *Policing, 6*(1), 4–15.

Shane, J. M. (2010). Performance management in police agencies: A conceptual framework. *Policing: An International Journal of Police Strategies & Management, 30*(1), 6–29.

Skogan, W. G. (2009). Concern about crime and confidence in the police: Reassurance or accountability? *Police Quarterly, 12*(3), 301–318.

Travis, A. (2014). Crime rate in England and Wales falls 15 % to its lowest level in 33 years. *The Guardian,* 24th April 2014.

Van Maanen, J. (1973). *Observations on the making of policemen.* Cambridge: Massachusetts Institute of Technology.

Waddington, P. A. J. (1999). Police (canteen) sub-culture: An appreciation. *British Journal of Criminology, 39*(2), 87–309.

Wankhade, P. (2011). Performance measurement and the UK emergency ambulance service: Unintended Consequences of the ambulance response time targets. *International Journal of Public Sector Management, 24*(5), 384–402.

Wankhade, P. & Barton, H. (2012). Conceptualising a police performance framework in an era of financial constraint. *Policing Today, 18*(3), 44–46.

Prof. Paresh Wankhade is the Professor of Leadership and Management at Edge Hill University Business School. He is a founding editor of International Journal of Emergency Services and is recognised as an expert in the field of emergency management. His research and publications focus on analyses of strategic leadership, organisational culture, organisational change and interoperability within the public services with a special focus on emergency services. His publications have contributed to inform debates around interoperability of public services and challenges faced by individual organisations.

Prof. David Weir is Visiting Professor at Edgehill University, and has held Chairs at several universities including Glasgow, Bradford, Liverpool Hope, UCS and SKEMA in France. He has worked with several police forces and has published extensively on risk management and undertook a major study with the Police Federation on the work of police sergeants in the UK. He has supervised more than sixty PhD theses on aspects of management and has written several books and many journal articles.

Chapter 2
Historical Perspective: British Policing and the Democratic Ideal

John G. D. Grieve

Introduction

The title of this piece is taken from Charles Reith's 1943 (Reith 1943) book whose writing and that of others has recently had a mixed press (Lentz and Chaires 2007). 'British' might be a slight misnomer on the part of this piece but it does consider Ireland and Scotland and their impact on Colquhoun, Peel and the first Commissioners of Police to the Metropolis. Part of the task here is to restore Reith's reputation to a wider audience. However the argument explores further back, further than the last 70 years, to 200 years ago. The participants here in this early account are seven. Later many more thinkers appear, before even the critical policing criminologists of in the mid twentieth Century. There are a complex network of tracks here to be mapped to understand the critiques and demands for reform of the twenty-first Century policing leadership, management and governance. This is not academic history, it is a practitioner's account of his predecessors but attempts to fulfil some of the requirements of the historian (for example MacMillan 2010, p. 5, 43) of orientation, considering context, asking questions, making connections and collecting and assessing evidence evidence. It is work in progress.

The chapter examines the roles of the policing philosophers John Stuart Mill and Jeremy Bentham, the magistrate Patrick Colquhoun, the politician Robert Peel, the administrator and legislator Edwin Chadwick, and the police practitioners, administrators, managers and leaders Charles Rowan and Richard Mayne, in charting a way. (It could have gone earlier to the Fielding brothers but does not consider ther highly important developments for lack of space.) The paper considers whether their thinking and research a century before him, informed Reith's arguments for British Policing Principles (Reith 1943, p. 4), and if it has any relevance to today.

J. G. D. Grieve (✉)
Portsmouth University, Portsmouth, UK
e-mail: jgdg@xob.demon.co.uk

© Springer International Publishing Switzerland 2015
P. Wankhade, D. Weir (eds.), *Police Services*, DOI 10.1007/978-3-319-16568-4_2

For example the reach of Bentham into the twenty-first Century has been, arguably, illustrated recently by the whistleblower on American and UK intelligence systems, Edward Snowden by his adoption of Bentham's coining of a 'Panopticon' as a way of describing the increased power of the state (see below and for example Harding (2014) which shows the philosophers continuing influence.

Recent changes in policing governance are significant, for example the 2012 arrival of the single person party political in many cases, elected Police and Crime Commissioners to replace the part elected 16 members, multi party bodies that were the Police Authorities (Brown 2014). These dated back to 1964 in current legislation but with a much earlier genesis. The Police and Crime Commissioners can be traced in part to American models (see Cohen below). Three American models are considered here and their relationship to the British model is considered.

Developing the theme of seeking the paths by which a British policing philosophy can be explored the chapter is particularly concerned with the twin imperatives from these early days; those of prevention and investigation and whether these conflict? This hypothesised tension might be taken to be further evidence of a crisis in democracy, in Reith's terms the democratic ideal, as well as the political debates of a crisis in policing leadership and management.[1]

The Early Thinkers and Practitioners of Policing

This piece does not claim that there is no role for politicians in determining policing strategy. On the contrary it is the task of policing to uphold the laws passed by politicians in Parliament. How that policing should be conducted is a matter in part for police practitioners and their leaders but they need to take account of the imperative for public support and the related issues of accountability and transparency. In a democracy the tactics and operations of the police need to be independent of the politicians, not least because sometimes the politicians may be the subject of police operations, just as the judiciary are required to be independent of the executive—the politicians in government in power and independent of everyone else. The police are accountable to the judiciary as they both uphold the law. Accountable in this sense means also giving an account of the exercise of their powers after the event to both the judiciary and politicians. Also they are accountable to the communities

---

[1] This paper distinguishes between the use of the words 'leadership' and 'management' in a way that many writers have pursued and about which there is still considerable debate. In short, because the issues can be discussed in volumes, leadership is about taking people somewhere they may not otherwise have gone and management is about the resources required, which includes the training and recruitment of those people. The related concept of 'command' of military origin but of considerable relevance to policing is a subset of leadership. (See the section on Elliot Cohen (2002) below). I am grateful to my colleagues both police and academic, with whom I have had many discussions on these topics. In particular I am very grateful Dr Andrew Fisher who falls into both categories and who continues to contribute to the material considered here not least about the relationship of Peel to Reith.

they were drawn from and so from earliest times needed to take into account the approval of many layers of the public; this was at the least through the jury system, in the criminal and civil courts and at Coroners Inquests dating back hundreds of years before Peel. That leads to thinking by policing leaders about the balance of independence and accountability in order to achieve public support (see for example Alderson (1979, 1984, 1998) for the detailed accounts of these imperatives, principles and developments over the years, written by a practitioner, academic and police philosopher).

Balancing difficult concepts is a task for philosophy. Critchley (1967) Stead (1977a) Ascoli (1979) Alderson (1998) all claim the influence of the Utilitarians on Peel and Chadwick and the early years of policing. Reith (1943) however does not cover their philosophy at all; he does however include both Bentham and Colquhoun in his 1952 book.

Jeremy Bentham (1748–1832) is arguable the thinker behind the emergence in the last 250 years of the police democratic ideal; the 'new' policing, what Alderson (1998) calls the 'good' or 'high' police balancing the issues raised by the need for public approval. He introduced thinking about this public approval (more generally called public or community confidence in the police today) and independence by articulating the greatest happiness (and least pain) principle, in part about the public good, founding the basis of a pleasure and pain calculus and it's relationship with miscarriages of justice. Indeed the words 'maximise' and 'minimise' were coined by him. The concept of a 'Panopticon' prison where the prisoners were visible at all times to ensure their good behaviour (and avoidance of pain inflicted by punishment for misbehaviour).[2] Bentham was a great influence on Colquhoun (Critchley 1967; Stead 1977a).

The philosopher who developed (indeed wrestled with) these ideas through the early years of policing was John Stuart Mill (1806–1873); his father was a friend of Bentham. He identified the issues at the heart of many debates about the public good, pleasure and pain and On Liberty the title of his most influential work. It was not for nothing that Peel wrote that liberty should not confused with being accosted by drunken women (sic), this is still relevant today as a recent bus journey on a Friday night in London showed. It is also evidence of the long shadows of philosophy that one of the most active pressure groups for police changes and reforms should be called Liberty at the time of writing (Critchley 1967; Stead 1977a, Alderson 1998).

Patrick Colquhoun (1745–1820) was a Magistrate at Thames Magistrates Court dealing with cases bought amongst others by the Thames Police patrolling the river through London. He was a close associate of Bentham, Stead writes that he admired

---

[2] This concept of constant visibility is what must have attracted Edward Snowden to the word Panopticon, in his case relating it to the constant visibility to the surveillance of the state through digital data. Continuing that thought of visibility another early example of intelligence is Bentham' close associate Colquhoun's (see below) knowledge of individual rioters behaviour and their identities. He made known to them his "forbearance" and admonished them to make good use of his forbearance an early example of preventive intelligence led policing (see Stead 1977b, p. 59) and even an early form of cautioning!

Colquhoun (Stead 1977b, p. 51). His Treatise on the Police of the Metropolis (1795) is a seminal work on policing and criminology not least on the criminology of policing. Colquhoun set about understanding the problem that police in its original sense, still to be found in the Police Instruction Books and web pages throughout the ages to this day, is some variation on "the arrangements made in civilised states to ensure the inhabitants keep the peace and obey the laws" (Alderson 1979, pp. 158–159). It is significant that the first Commissioners were Magistrates—that is Justices of the Peace.

Colquhoun made a detailed record, gathered data, defined his terms, analysed the data, explored motivation, came to conclusions and made recommendations. Not surprisingly, given what he did, he described policing as a new science. His definition of police is interesting but slightly more complex than that given above. It is "all those regulations in a country which apply to the comfort, convenience and safety of the inhabitants" (Stead 1977b, p. 51; Reith 1952, pp. 136–149). It is suggested that regulations means more than just those set up under legislation. Which definition aptly describes the police tasks today. Colquhoun is the architect of the preventive paradigm in policing, the prevention of crime as the primary object of the wider definition of police, including prevention by detection and punishment.

Peel offered his thoughts generally on how the 'new' Police should act in a debate in Parliament on 28th February 1828; he outlined what he had seen in Paris and Scotland[3]. He thought they should epitomise—(that the Police Officer as a) "Public Officer for that purpose, who apart from malice and private considerations, is bound to execute his duty with impartiality and firmness." (Parliamentary Debate 28.2.1828 paragraph 795 MEPO 7/1 PRO). Impartiality and fairness is the foundation of the independence of chief officers and all who hold the Office of Constable under the Crown in the British model.

Robert Peel certainly did not write out or articulate any list of policing principles that resembles Reith (1943, p. 3) in their entirety. Or if he did we have not found them. It is disappointing to trawl through the Public Records Office Peel papers and the early Metropolitan Police letter books (MEPO). The records are of politics and drunkenness. That is Peel's politics and police and public drunkenness. There are accounts of recruitment and pay and the general character and backgrounds of police recruits. There is an illuminating letter (cited in Hurd 2007, p. 106) on the artisan nature of the tasks that Peel was proposing. There is no outline of principles of how policing was to be done nor an overall strategy; that has to be inferred from the later correspondence and first police instruction books. The issue here is not that Peel wrote the Principles but what is the evidence that he believed in some or all of the values they espoused? The two first Commissioners Rowan and Mayne turned Peels legislation into practical instructions for the 'new' police in the spring and summer of 1829 (see Times Newspaper 25.9.1829 pages 2 and 3). By autumn of

---

[3] Not it should be noted Ireland as he is often described as getting his thinking from his experiences there. He goes on to cite his learning about the nature and behaviour of policing in London, Liverpool, Manchester, Glasgow, (and eventually) Dublin and Edinburgh ("Parliamentary" Debate 28.2.1828 paragraph 788).

that year they were ready. The combination of the disciplines of military, law, philosophy and politics has cast long shadows on the path policing governance, management and leadership has followed (Reith 1952; Critchley 1967; Stead 1977a; Alderson 1979, 1984, 1998).

Charles Rowan was an army officer, trained by Robert Craufurd in the Napoleonic Peninsular campaigns. He was a staff officer who wrote well and was probably involved in the writing of a forgotten early nineteenth Century treatise on the policing of military camps (Fletcher 1991). The military paradigm is at the heart of many debates about policing and police leadership down the ages to this day. Rowan drafted the initial Instruction Book that outlined the demeanour, tasks and duties of the Office of Constable under the Crown that pulled together all the good in what had gone before. Making sure that the duties were conducted in the style that Peel desired was a leadership and management task from the outset that Rowan described to his Superintendents—their badge a Crown being the Warrant Officer's not the Major's, further proof of the artisan nature of policing that Peel had desired (Times Newspaper 25.9.1829 pages 2 and 3; Reith 1952; Critchley 1967; Stead 1977a; Alderson (1979), (1984) and (1998)). The nature of policing, it's demeanour and tasks remain a management and leadership task to this day.

In a famous letter (cited in Hurd 2007, p. 106) Peel had written that he did not want 'gentlemen' (and presumably would not want ladies today)[4] in his 'new' police. His reasons are arguably mixed; control of the working classes and non working classes he anticipated would be better achieved by artisans and their leaders from the same class albeit with an officer and a gentleman as the first Commissioners. This patronising and class based issue remains the basis for some attitudes to the police and from some of the police themselves to this day.[5]

Richard Mayne, Rowan's co commissioner initially and then sole incumbent epitomises the legal paradigm in policing, Mayne had been a Magistrate in Ireland. Whilst Rowan was outlining the tasks and demeanour of the new police Mayne drafted the legal basis on which the police officers' powers rested. (Reith 1952; Critchley 1967; Stead 1977a,). Another abiding leadership and management task to this day.

It is worth remembering that Rowan and Mayne were both appointed as Justices of the Peace, a quasi judicial role retained until late in the twentieth Century by Metropolitan Police Commissioners.

---

[4] See footnote 1.

[5] A senior officer said to the author of this paper in 1986 that "policing was a working man's job that had been hijacked by intellectuals" he might have added, based on the authors assessment of his mindset "and women". But he did not. This is not an attitude the author approves, nor holds as either helpful or correct.

Charles Reith and the 'Not Peelian' Principles

Charles Reith does not claim that Peel wrote the 9 Principles that he recorded at the start of his account of policing and democracy (Reith 1943, pp. 3–4). Peel's name does not appear at all in Reith's first chapter and when it does appear 11 pages in, it is in the context of "party tactics and political manoeuvring "(Reith 1943, p. 11). Reith (1952, p. 139) considers that "Although his contribution... was an essential one, it was very small in comparison with what was contributed by each of the others. The share of fame that was allotted to him by historians was unfair." What Reith is arguing for is longer tradition and public support for order and peace (most of the time) and for its role in national unity, if not for public support for the actual establishment of a public or new uniformed police.

So the nine principles of police as articulated by Reith are separate from Peel:

1. To prevent crime and disorder, as an alternative to their repression by military force and severity of legal punishment.
2. To recognise always that the power of the police to fulfil their functions and duties is dependent on public approval of their existence, actions and behaviour, and on their ability to secure and maintain public respect.
3. To recognise always that to secure and maintain the respect and approval of the public means also the securing of the willing co-operation of the public in the task of securing observance of laws.
4. To recognise always that the extent to which the co-operation of the public can be secured diminishes, proportionately, the necessity of the use of physical force and compulsion for achieving police objectives.
5. To seek and to preserve public favour, not by pandering to public opinion, but by constantly demonstrating absolutely impartial service to Law, in complete independence of policy, and without regard to the justice or injustice of the substance of individual laws; by ready offering of individual service and friendship to all members of the public without regard to their wealth or social standing; by ready exercise of courtesy and friendly good humour; and by ready offering of individual sacrifice in protecting and preserving life.
6. To use physical force only when the exercise of persuasion, advice and warning is found to be insufficient to obtain public co-operation to an extent necessary to secure observance of law or to restore order; and to use only the minimum degree of physical force which is necessary on any particular occasion for obtaining a police objective.
7. To maintain at all times a relationship with the public that gives reality to the historic tradition that the police are the public and that the public are the police; the police being only members of the public who are paid to give full time attention to duties which are incumbent on every citizen, in the interests of community welfare and existence.
8. To recognise always the need for strict adherence to police-executive functions, and to refrain from even seeming to usurp the powers of the judiciary of avenging individuals or the State, and of authoritatively judging guilt and punishing the guilty.
9. To recognise always that the test of police efficiency is the absence of crime and disorder, and not the visible evidence of police action in dealing with them.
(Reith 1943, pp. 3–4)

What follows is an attempt to anchor these principles in the past and apply them to today.

Clive Emsley said in a presentation recently that the so called Peelian Principles may not have been articulated by Robert Peel but they seemed like good ideas and most policing thinkers today would probably sign up to them[6]. There is evidence of that from both sides of the Atlantic and across the Irish Sea. Peel may not have listed them but there is much in the public record that supports the contention that he may have supported the thinking behind versions of Reith's 9 Principles (Reith 1943, p. 34).

Some Later Usage of the 'Not Peelian' Principles

The Americans and their thinking about police reform and the democratic ideal produced the police practitioner academics August Vollmer and (MacNamara 1977) his protégée O.W. Wilson. (Vollmer 1936; Carte and Carte (1977)). Their work and its influence illustrates from the US experiences in 1930s what Steve Savage (2007) called the trade winds of policing thinking that crossed both the Irish Sea and the Atlantic. These trade winds might also be seen as sea ways, another form of path to be followed. They may help in preparing a map of ideas and values in policing. Wilson wrote about the British Police model and a review of Reith's studies so he was well aware of the non Peelian Principles (Wilson 1950a, b, c).

Tom Critchley a distinguished UK civil servant was the secretary to the 1964 Royal Commission and subsequently wrote a history of policing (Critchley 1967, 1977). Paying tribute to the scholarship of Radzinowicz (1956) he discusses at length the related roles of Bentham and Colquhoun in establishing the primary task of police as prevention.

The work of Philip John Stead on the pioneers and reformers of policing (Stead 1977b) had a profound impact on the thinking explored here whilst he was at the Police Staff College Bramshill in the 1970s and later in the USA at John Jay University New York in the 1980s; the Staff College is a casualty of the contemporary politicisation of police. The Metropolitan Police library that Reith had used was another casualty. Stead covered each of the founding fathers. Tom Critchley was his contributor on Colquhoun (Critchley 1977).

David Ascoli writing to celebrate 150 years of the Metropolitan Police in 1979 also considers the related roles of the founding fathers (Ascoli 1979) dedicating his book to Rowan and Mayne and their contribution to the subsequent history of policing.

In the follow up to Lord Scarman's third Inquiry, the one into the Brixton Disorders (Scarman 1981) [7]another American model that of Lubans and Edgar (1979) appeared. This was a variation on the theories of management by objectives applied as a complete structure of policing. Policing by objectives appeared in UK police

---

[6] Emsley (2014) this was at a workshop organised by Professor Jennifer Brown of the academic thinking behind The Lord Stevens Inquiry into Policing for a Better Britain (Stevens (2014) Brown Ed (2014)).

[7] Lord Scarman conducted three public inquiries. Red Lion Square. Northern Ireland. The Brixton Disorders. All of these could be argued to have a relevance to this discussion.

managers bookshelves in the early 1980s as part of advice on UK reforms from the US Police Foundation and in particular research and recommendations from John Eck on volume crimes. Stephen Savage's study of the history of the twentieth and early twenty-first Century reforms helps explore the issues, particularly the role of the police themselves on reform from within, and sets the context and interpretation (Savage 2007). Robert Reiner's (2000) hugely influential 'The Politics of Police' was a major contribution to understanding the context and environment of policing governance. He describes the Principles as Reithian and "a significant reference point for British police thinking" (Reiner 2000, p. 24).

About this time Robert Fleming aided by Hugh Miller made a fly on the wall extensive TV documentary series which was to be the forerunner of many to come, they accompanied it with a near 400 page book (Fleming and Miller 1994) which intriguingly both denies and confirms the thesis presented here. They interviewed dozens of senior Metropolitan Police Service officers from the Commissioner downwards. On the one hand there is no mention of Peel or any of the founding fathers by name; on the other hand their ideas are everywhere. The principles, 50 years after Reith, seem to have been ingested. There are fortunately a number of women interviewed. For example "the police are the public and the public are the police" principle as epitomised by *Crimestoppers* (Fleming and Miller 1994, p. 261), the importance of prevention in this instance by investigation, detection and intervention before the crime is committed—in this case armed robbery—arrested by Flying Squad officers in a perfect illustration of Colquhoun's preventive police (Fleming and Miller 1994, p. 101).

Robert Adlam and Peter Villiers both former academic tutors at the UK Police Staff College produced a useful volume of contributions on rethinking police leadership for the arrival of the twenty-first Century (Adlam and Villiers 2003). They derive some principles which form an interesting commentary on those prepared by Reith.

Sir Patrick Sheehy was asked by Kenneth Clark then conservative Home Secretary to look at police management structures and conditions of service (Sheehy 1993; Brain 2010; Savage 2007).

Down the years many attempts were made by different governments to reintroduce military values into police leadership.[8] for example the scheme by Lord Trenchard to introduce an officer class in the 1930s. A different American military model was explored by a later conservative government. Policy Exchange a conservative think tank, asked Eliot Cohen an American academic to adapt some of the thinking in his book about the military leadership and politicians, Supreme Command, (Cohen 2002) to the relationship between politicians and police leaders. The book used the examples of Lincoln, Clemenceau, Churchill and Ben Gurion to

---

[8] A recent Commissioner to the Metropolis once told the author of the comment made by a very senior soldier to him "the trouble with the police is that they have no honour." Perhaps he meant they are neither gentlemen nor ladies. The artisan model of policing was alive and well in some officers' messes. Another recent commentator on an exclusive officers military club claimed "they did not want Plod in here" they were referring to counter terrorist specialists.

illustrate the different ways politicians might interact with at the least and control at the maximum their military leadership:

- President Abraham Lincoln writing a letter to his military commander Ulysses S. Grant during the American Civil War:
- The French Premier Clemenceau visiting his front line troops and their commanders in the First World War following the mutinies of 1917 regularly one day a week
- Wartime Prime Minister Winston Churchill's methods of asking difficult questions of his military leaders
- Israeli Prime Minister Ben Gurion's thinking and workshops called 'seminars' because of the intellectual rigour he demanded. His raw materials were the Hagannah and other guerrilla forces that he forged together for the creation of the Israeli Defence Forces. He created a disciplined body from the disparate guerrilla armies that had fought the British during the League of Nations/UN Mandate in Palestine.

What these each have in common are that they are about supreme political command at times of grave national danger in wartime. Political intervention was not just a possibility but an imperative, a necessity. How can that be compared with the situation of police reforms? Can it be argued that a situation in policing is analogous outside of where the politician's judge there is a grave national danger? One possible exceptional answer might be the example of some periods in Northern Ireland which led for example to the second Lord Scarman Inquiry, where the situation especially the alleged exhaustion of the RUC was judged so grave that the Army was deployed, as Military Aid to the Civil Powers (MACP) (Brain 2010, p. 14).

"The Last Great Unreformed Public Body"?

Finally this section seeks to understand the influence, if any, of the history of non Peelian Principles in changes in police governance and management in the twenty-first century.

Four sets of recent papers, the first by former Chief Constable Peter Neyroud, the next by Sir Denis O'Connor then Her Majesty's Chief Inspector of Constabulary and two linked ones by lawyer and former rail regulator now Her Majesty's Chief Inspector of Constabulary Tom Winsor, the last by former Commissioner Lord John Stevens and Professor Jennifer M. Brown explore the issues of policing in an age of austerity and increased political and media intervention. The content and commentaries on these might illustrate the relevance and significance of the early thinkers to today's issues and reforms.

Some critical commentators on the reforms that are apparently required, for example Nick Hopkins and Sandra Lavelle (2014, p. 15) consider the arguments that this period of extreme reform and proposed further reform of policing as alleged by some could have been driven by party politics not least by the current Prime Minister[9] and also as alleged could be political revenge for the alleged ill judged police investigation and inquiries in the Palace of Westminster into Damien Green MP[10] (albeit the investigation had been started at the bequest of another political party, the Government at the time as is largely forgotten now) and the MP's expenses scandals (which was generated by media revelations in the Daily Telegraph).

Peter Neyroud a former Chief Constable and Tom Winsor later HMCIC, are both, intentionally or otherwise driving Government sponsored radical reform programs that navigates the landscape of a political agenda in an age of austerity; they seem uninterested in the past and in tradition. Neyroud (2011) is concerned with the paths and preparation for leadership, indeed for supreme command though not on the Cohen model. The limited references Neyroud cites are American though.

Sir Denis O'Connor was explicit in the role he identified for the founding fathers in the British Policing Model that he recommended be the foundation of policing. In two hard hitting HMCIC Reports (Her Majesty's Chief Inspectorate of Constabulary) he reminded the service of its origins and the contemporary relevance and significance of the non Peelian Principles (HMCIC 2009a, b).

Winsor (2012) considered the recruitment and conditions of service of police. In particular he reintroduced the officers and gentlemen debate by proposing and then driving direct entry at Superintendent level, most commentators then assumed this was to mean officers at the conclusion of their military careers.

Former Metropolitan Police Commissioner Lord John Stevens and Professor Jennifer Brown from LSE in 2012 and 2013 drove a number of projects academic and pragmatic that supported a Government Opposition party political alternative to the twenty-first Century Government driven reforms. They commissioned a wide ranging review of policing (Stevens 2014; Brown (2014)). The Commission examined the relevance of the 'non Peelian Principles', in considerable detail and seems to offer radical reforms but in the sense of seeking new ways to support traditional values in policing like those expressed by Reith in the non Peelian Principles. Their book of academic papers to support the commission's report contains a number of contributions which offer insight for the contemporary relevance (Brown 2014).

Conclusion

This chapter has suggested that in the twenty-first Century there is more to be ingested still from the 'non Peelian' Principles. There is much debate about the nature of states and their structures and powers and that if that might be a crisis in the democratic ideal then that crisis underpins any account of a crisis in policing, and also underpins any crisis in policing governance, leadership and management.

---

[9] David Cameron Prime Minister at the time of writing was part of Kenneth Clarke's association to Patrick Sheehy's Review of Policing.

[10] Damien Green MP was alleged to have been involved in the leakage of documents from a minister's office whilst his party was in opposition. At the time of writing he had just finished a period as Minister for Policing in the Home Office.

Reith's versions of the 9 Principles owe much to the founding fathers but also to the much earlier attempts to keep the peace and obey the law. What Reith describes as the tradition of the British Police and the Democratic Ideal stretches back to before Bentham and Colquhoun let alone Peel. This is not to deny Bentham's, Colquhoun's or Peel's influence on Rowan and Mayne and their articulation of the first philosophy, strategy, policy, practices and processes of the public or new police.

Peel deserves much of the credit for the practical, political but essential role in the development of the emerging framework, even if not the precise labelling of them as Peel's Principles that he has sometimes been given. But he should be given the credit as an artificer[11] building on what had been begun earlier rather than as a completely original thinker as Douglas Hurd's work advises us (Hurd 2007). He made the democratic ideal of British Police begin to happen. Reith's articulation remains helpful as an ideal. The Principles, ancient though they are in origin, have relevance and resonance today. They are like stones on old footpaths that were trodden by many before us. They are still markers on a path to be followed. The path is abandoned by leadership, management or command, whether supreme or operational, at the peril of contemporary democracy.

References

Adlam, R., & Villiers, P. (2003). *Police leadership in the 21st century*. Winchester: Waterside Press.
Alderson, J. (1979). *Policing freedom*. Plymouth: Macdonald and Evans.
Alderson, J. (1984). *Law and disorder*. London: Hamish Hamilton.
Alderson, J. (1998). *Principled policing*. Winchester: Waterside Press.
Ascoli, D. (1979). *The queen's peace*. London: Hamish Hamiltion.
Brain, T. (2010). *A history of policing in England and Wales from 1974: A turbulent journey*. Oxford: Oxford University Press.
Brown, J. (Ed.). (2014). *The future of policing*. London: Routledge.
Carte, G. E., & Carte, E. (1977). O.W. Wilson: Police theory in action. In P. J. Stead (Ed.), *Pioneers in policing*. Montclair: Patterson Smith.
Cohen, E. (2002). *Supreme command*. New York: Simon and Schuster.
Colqhoun, P. (1795). *A treatise on the police of the metropolis*. London.
Critchley, T. A. (1967). *A history of the police in England and Wales*. London: Constable and Company.
Critchley, T. A. (1977). Peel, rowan and mayne: The British model of police. In P. J. Stead (Ed.), *Pioneers in policing*. Montclair: Patterson Smith.
Emsley, C. (2009). *The great British bobby*. London: Quercus.
Emsley, C. (2014). Peel's principles, police principles. In J. Brown (Ed.), *The future of policing* (pp. 11–22). London: Routledge.
Fleming, R., & Miller, H. (1994). *Scotland yard*. London: Michael Joseph.
Fletcher, I. (1991). *Craufurd's light brigade*. London: Spellmount.

---

[11] A contemporary analogy for the work of Bentham, Colquhoun, Peel, Rowan and Mayne, Chadwick and Mill in London and beyond might be the innovators who gathered at Stanford University and migrated to Silicon Valley in the 1980s. It is perhaps also relevant that Vollmer and Wilson in a later age came from California.

Harding, L. (2014). *The Snowden files*. London: Guardian Books.

HMCIC. (2009a). *Adapting to protest—nurturing the British model of policing*. 25.11.2009. Her Majesty's Chief Inspector of Policing. Home Office, London.

HMCIC. (2009b). *Adapting to protest—facilitating peaceful protest*. 25.11.2009. Her Majesty's Chief Inspector of Policing. Home Office, London.

Hopkins, N., & Laville, S. (15 February 2014). 'We haven't changed in 100 years': Disarray in the ranks leaves union hierarchy in crisis. *Guardian Newspaper, 15*. London.

Hurd, D. (2007). *Robert Peel*. London: Weidenfeld and Nicolson.

Lentz, S. A., & Chaires, R. H. (2007). The invention of Peel's principles: A study of policing 'textbook' history. *Journal of Criminal Justice, 35*, 69–79.

Lubans, V. A., & Edgar, J. M. (1979). *Policing by objectives: A handbook for improving police management*. Connecticut: Hartford Social Development Corporation.

MacMillan, M. (2010). *The uses and abuses of history*. London: Profile Books.

MacNamara, D. E. J. (1977). August Vollmer: The vision of police professionalism. In P. J. Stead (Ed.), *Pioneers in policing*. Montclair: Patterson Smith.

Neyroud, P. (2011). *Review of police leadership and training*. London: Home Office.

Radzinowicz, L. (1956). *A history of the English criminal law and it's administration from 1750*. London.

Reiner, R. (2000). *The politics of the police* (3rd ed.). Oxford: Oxford University Press.

Reith, C. (1943). *British policing and the democratic ideal*. London: Oxford University Press.

Reith, C. (1952). *The blind eye of history*. London: Faber.

Savage, S. (2007). *Police reform. Forces for change*. Oxford: Oxford University Press.

Scarman, L. (1981). The *Brixton disorders: Report of an inquiry*. London: HMSO.

Sheehy, P. (1993). *Inquiry into police responsibilities and rewards*. London: HMSO.

Stead, P. J. (1977a). *Pioneers in policing*. Montclair: Patterson Smith.

Stead, P. J. (1977b). Patrick Colquhoun-Preventive police. In P. J. Stead (Ed.), *Pioneers in policing*. Montclair: Patterson Smith.

Stevens, J. (2014). *Policing for a better Britain*. Independent Commission into the Future of Policing. Essex: Lord Stevens and the Anton Group.

Vollmer, A. (1936 reprinted 1969). *The police and modern society*. California: University of California.

Wilson, O. W. (1950a). *Police administration*. New York: McGraw Hill.

Wilson, O. W. (1950b). Review of Charles Reith: Short history of the British police. *Journal of Criminal Law & Criminology, 40*(5), 675–677.

Wilson, O. W. (1950c). The British police. *Journal of Criminal Law & Criminology, 40*(5), 637–650.

Winsor, T. P. (2012). *Independent review of police officer and staff remuneration and conditions*. London: TSO. Command 8325.

Prof. John G. D. Grieve CBE. QPM. BA (Hons). M.Phil. joined the Metropolitan Police in 1966 at Clapham and served as a police officer and detective throughout London, in every role from undercover officer to policy chair for over 37 years before retiring in 2002. His duties involved the Drugs, Flying, Robbery and Murder Squads senior investigator. He was also the borough commander at Bethnal Green and head of training at Hendon Police College and was the first Director of Intelligence for the Metropolitan Police. He was appointed as one of four Commissioners of the International Independent Monitoring Commission for some aspects of the peace process in Northern Ireland in 2003 by the UK Government until 2011. He is a Senior Research Fellow at University of Portsmouth and Professor Emeritus at London Metropolitan University. He currently chairs the MoJ/HO Independent Advisory Group on Hate Crime and advises a number of policing bodies including on cultural matters. He has written extensively on policing matters including leadership and creativity.

Part II
Context of Policing

Chapter 3
Quo Vadis: A New Direction for Police Leadership Through Community Engagement?

Andrew C. Fisher and John M. Phillips

Introduction: A Service in Peril

The police service is in crisis. What that crisis is about is in plain view. What is not so clear is why it is so. What is even less clear is how the crisis will be resolved.

Management gurus in the 1990s thought it insightful to juxtapose the Chinese idiom for 'crisis' as meaning either 'peril', or 'opportunity'. A quarter of a century later a sense of peril is very strong but it is far from clear what there is opportunity for, and where the police service might go to find it. To parody Sir Edward Grey, British Foreign Secretary in 1914, 'the [police] lamps are going out all over...'.

This chapter seeks to examine what the nature of the crisis might be, briefly how the police service has got to this stage of organisational peril, and then to suggest a new direction for its leadership that will take it out of tired leadership initiatives modelled on heroic and messianic panaceas for crisis.

The nature of the problems facing the police service in England and Wales are multi-faceted. They are, at the very least, political, fiscal, structural, cultural, and societal. In the midst of them, and running through them all, might be a leadership crisis.

At the turn of the century, the International Association of Chiefs of Police considered the future in these terms, 'Perhaps the biggest challenge facing police executives of the twenty-first century will be to develop police organizations that can effectively recognise, relate and assimilate the global shifts in culture, technology and information. Changing community expectations, workforce values, technological power, governmental arrangements, policing philosophies, and ethical standards

A. C. Fisher (✉) · J. M. Phillips
Liverpool Hope University, Liverpool, UK
e-mail: fishera@hope.ac.uk

J. M. Phillips
e-mail: phillij@hope.ac.uk

© Springer International Publishing Switzerland 2015
P. Wankhade, D. Weir (eds.), *Police Services,* DOI 10.1007/978-3-319-16568-4_3

are but a sample of the forces that must be understood and constructively managed by the current and incoming generation of chief executives' (IACP 1999, p. 1). In the traditional manner, responsibility for dealing with the challenges was laid at the door of the leader in chief.

The focus on leadership of the police service persists, but since the formation of the Coalition government in 2010 there has been a shift at Westminster in the ideological and political stance towards the police. It was signalled by the Home Secretary in 2010 when Theresa May set a new agenda for the police: 'I couldn't be any clearer about your mission: it isn't a thirty-point plan; it is to cut crime. No more, and no less'. It was followed by proposed policy changes across the structure of policing derived from the Winsor Report (2011) affecting pay and conditions, and laying the basis for fundamental shifts, like direct entry at senior officer level, in the way policing was led and managed. The political wave swept into the local accountability of 41 police services with the creation of Police and Crime Commissioners (PCC) to be elected to oversee the provincial forces, London's Metropolitan Police excepted. Local accountability saw the old Police Authorities swept away as PCCs provided a singular locus for Chief Constables to report to. Politicians are now assuming the role of correctives of the police service rather than agents.

To the political are added fiscal problems. The 2010 Comprehensive Spending Review initiated by the Coalition foreshadowed extensive cuts in the public service, and especially in the budgets of the police throughout England and Wales. From 2010 to 2014 spending on the police was to be reduced by 20 % and, in 2013 a further cap was announced, with additional cuts of around 6 % from 2015. The impact was immediate and the debate about where those cuts might fall and what the consequences for the effectiveness of policing and cutting crime might be gathered a quick pace. The principle of Best Value, and the three Es of public service funding from the 1980s were as relevant as ever, as 'economy, effectiveness and efficiency' were applied to policing, whilst a debate about where the front line of policing was, and how it might be protected for the sake of the public, opened up. With the cuts, the onus upon the police to provide an effective and efficient service has grown heavier.

It can be further argued that the problems underlying the crisis are structural. The size of the Metropolitan Police alone has led some (Loader 2014) to question whether in fact it is governable. The notion of its 32 boroughs as autonomous units lies uneasily with the accusations that they are laws unto themselves, 'organised anarchies' as Cohen et al. (1972) suggested universities were. The charge is that there is limited co-ordination and integration, that policing south of the Thames is different in character from policing north of the river, that rivalries and jealousies within the Met's sections and departments inhibit its effectiveness, and its relationships with forces outside London smack of a perceived superiority and arrogance. The wider structural picture is made up of 43 forces in England and Wales. The possibility of force mergers has come and gone with regularity, but Scotland now has, since 2013, just one force, and some expect Wales to follow suit soon.

There is reason to believe the problems are cultural. The so-called 'Plebgate' affair in 2012, involving a Minister of the Crown, Andrew Mitchell, and forcing his resignation from the government, exposed allegations of conspiracy, crimes and misdemeanours by members of the Police Federation, and no doubt, were there such an accusation as 'bringing the service into disrepute' that too could have been levelled against it. As it was, an Independent Report (Normington 2014), into the Police Federation, established by its own hands, suggested a tranche of reforms, and led the chair of the Federation, Steve Williams, to declare, 'It's fair to say we haven't helped ourselves. The federation has been around for 100 years but we haven't changed'. The Plebgate affair might suggest a wider, cultural malaise. The Times headlined in November 2013, 'We regularly fiddle crime numbers, admit police' (Ford 2014). In January 2014 police crime figures lost their credibility. The UK Statistics Authority removed the National Statistics quality assurance mark from all crime figures supplied by the police, because, it said, the Office for National Statistics did not have sufficient confidence in the quality of the data. The parliamentary Public Administration Committee had heard from one Met officer in December 2013 that the emphasis on hitting performance targets had led to police fiddling the figures, and that this was now 'an ingrained part of policing culture'. Lord Stevens, the former Met Commissioner, told the Home Affairs Select Committee in January 2014, that officers in one force had told him that massaging crime statistics was 'the biggest scandal coming our way'.

Elements of a corrosive culture appear to surface regularly. In a Her Majesty's Inspectorate of Constabulary (HMIC) report into the police's handling of domestic abuse victims, many of the police's failings were blamed on the culture and values of individual officers. 'HMIC is concerned about the poor attitudes that some police officers display towards victims of domestic abuse...Victims told us that they were frequently not taken seriously, that they felt judged and that some officers demonstrated a considerable lack of empathy and understanding,' (HMIC 2014a).

To exacerbate matters, the problems increasingly appear to lie in the police's relationship with society. The Peelian principles, invoked as the basis of British policing by public consent, may be known to few, even within the police service, but the attitude to the police of whole sections of society, by geography and social class, has been shaken by a series of policing scandals stretching back over a quarter of a century. These are not simply historical phenomena as their disclosure and the implications they have given rise to are significant elements in the current crisis. The 1962 Royal Commission on The Police reported: "No less than 83 % of those interviewed professed great respect for the police, 16 % said they had mixed feelings, and only 1 % said they had little or no respect." Public opinion polls today register public confidence at about 66 % (Maybin 2014). At only two-thirds support, public trust in the police is low as a succession of black marks is set against the police record, with a suggestion that first contacts with police officers actually reduces confidence (Bradford et al. 2009). Within the last couple of years the role of several police forces in the Hillsborough football stadium tragedy in 1989, and in subsequent police enquiries, has led to criminal investigation into their conduct. The behaviour of the police during the national miners' strikes of the 1980s, and at Orgreave in Yorkshire in particular in 1984, has been re-examined against charges of conspiracy, cover-up and perverting the course of justice. The shooting by a police officer of Mark Duggan in north London in 2011 sparked a summer of riots and disturbances across the capital but also in towns and cities outside London. The 'summer of discontent' (Briggs 2013) suggested a diminished relationship with and respect for the police. The investigation into the Stephen Lawrence murder in 1992, and the ensuing enquiry into that investigation, the Macpherson Report 1999, have been shown to be quite incomplete as revelation upon revelation of undercover deception, of allegations of police corruption, and of perpetuated institutional racism shake the foundations of the Metropolitan Police. The undercover role of the police and the SDS (Special Demonstration Squad) of the Metropolitan Police, have extended the accusations to institutionalised sexism for the way the police have sought to frustrate claims by women deceived into sexual relations by undercover officers (Boffey 2014). In this regard Lord Macdonald, a former Director of Public Prosecutions, accused the police of engendering a 'culture of conceit'.

As the crises mounted for the Metropolitan Police, in March 2014 and following the publication of a further report into the police handling of the Lawrence investigation, by Mark Ellison QC, Sir Bernard Hogan Howe, its Commissioner, declared it to be 'a devastating report for the Metropolitan Police and one of the worst days that I have seen as a police officer'. He concluded 'The Metropolitan Police will not regain lost trust without honesty, openness and transparency', but for Lord Macdonald 'policing was now scraping the bottom'. Indeed within days it got worse for the Commissioner. Appearing before the Commons Home Affairs Committee, committee chair Keith Vaz told Sir Bernard, "Normally I find you very reassuring to this committee. I am afraid I don't think we are reassured at the moment." Asked if there should be an inquiry into 'the Met as a whole', Sir Bernard said: 'No. There's no need. It's absolute nonsense. We are doing very well'. But Vaz announced a full parliamentary inquiry into the 'structure, governance and culture' of the Met. This followed the Home Secretary commissioning HMIC to include in its inspection into police integrity and leadership a specific examination of the anti-corruption capability of police forces, including force professional standards departments (HMIC 2014b).

But for all that things are bad for the Metropolitan Police and its Commissioner, the key problem is public confidence. The 'Plebgate' affair rocked public confidence: if a minister of the Crown could be conspired against what chance did ordinary members of the public have? Writing in the Daily Telegraph in October 2013, the Chief Constable of Avon and Somerset Constabulary, acknowledged the scale of the problem, in that 'the reaction [to the 'Mitchell cloud'] we have all seen (and it is intense) comes not from that ground level, but from an educated middle class: people who read, and write for, broadsheet newspapers and listen to the Today programme'. And for those people this is huge. And it matters. Many are asking themselves for the first time in their lives. 'Can I really trust the Police?' (Gargan 2013).

Finally one may consider the systemic crisis as part of the structural problems some critics point to within the police service or one may see it as a crisis of leadership, and leadership at every level throughout the police service. One Chief Constable has been dismissed, in Cleveland in 2013, as was the Deputy there; others, in Gwent and in Avon and Somerset, went with the coming of the PCC, and vacancies remained unfilled and failed to attract the expected number of applicants in several areas throughout 2012–2013. Caerphilly MP Wayne David said it was "not surprising" that the number of applicants for the vacant position of Chief Constable at Gwent Police was limited (Sanders 2013). Leadership of the police service may be perceived as something of a poisoned chalice. And if the leadership at the top is not right, this must make it harder for effective and ethical leadership to permeate the service at every level.

When faced by scandal and crisis, apology has become the institutional response. Past mistakes are admitted and deeply regretted. A firm purpose of amendment is announced, and then the next scandal breaks. This systemic weakness and failure to learn are the points at which the police lose moral authority and legitimacy. The consequences of this must be enormous. Adlam (2002) refers to a 'moral panic rationality' when questions arise as to the fairness, consistency and image of the police, with this resulting in its legitimacy being questioned.

In his first annual report (HMIC 2014b) to the Home Secretary, HM Chief Inspector of Constabulary, Tom Winsor, citing Hillsborough, Orgreave, Lawrence and its aftermath, 'Plebgate', and the SDS, admitted that 'controversies and revelations of a serious and negative nature in relation to the conduct of some police officers, both past and present, have hurt public confidence in the police' (para 8) and that 'loss of trust in the police is corrosive to the heart of the British model of policing by consent (para 78)…The police service has been damaged, but it is certainly not broken.' Significantly, and perhaps all too predictably, he added, 'It is primarily the responsibility of the leadership of the police to repair the damage which has been done' (para 8). This may be the crisis at its core, because to assert a leadership responsibility for its resolution gives insight into neither the form of leadership intended nor the strategy for the leadership to adopt.

False Illusions

The present is the product of the past. One can therefore ask how far past leadership behaviours and strategies have contributed to the current crisis or sense of crisis.

Up to the 1980s it is reasonable to suggest that police forces (sic) in general and chief constables in particular exercised a high degree of autonomy and control in both what they did and how they did it. Police authorities exercised an accounting check and balance, but few conflicts and controversies between them and their police chiefs pepper the period after the Second World War. Williams (2003) argues that in this period the Home Office constantly sought to remove police forces from local control, and local political influence, and that scandal and corruption were the excuse, in the Police Act 1964, for a system in which 'the Chief Constable was accountable for executive decisions to the Home Secretary in practice, and nobody in theory'.

The landscape changed in the 1980s. The Thatcher governments implemented a New Public Management (Hood 1991), the cornerstones of which continued to

apply for the next 30 years under successive Conservative and New Labour governments. The principles of NPM, characterised as 'accountability, responsibility, and
responsiveness' challenged the public services to match the best practices of the
private sector. In this way the sought-for modernisation of the public services, their
increased effectiveness and efficiency, would be secured with greater economy. A
core feature of NPM was described by Osborne and Gaebler (1992) as a separation
between 'steering' and 'rowing' in the delivery of services. In other words, central
government provided strategic direction in terms of budget and policy (steering)
while other agencies, including the police, were given responsibility for the delivery of services (rowing) (Reiner 2010; Savage 2007b; Golding and Savage 2008).
This has been described as 'governing at a distance' resulting in central government
being able to penetrate parts of policing that they had not previously been able to
access or influence, such as the day to day operation of discretion (Reiner 2010;
Savage 2007b). This type of 'power beyond the state' is a characteristic of political
action being practised 'at a distance' (Miller and Rose 1990) and, perhaps more
importantly, the government was able to exercise its authority over that most pre-
cious of commodities—resources, while vesting the responsibility for increases in
resources on the police themselves through achieving performance targets.

Ferlie et al. (1996) describe 'New Public Management in Action' as involving
the introduction into public services of the 'three Ms': markets, managers and measurement. It ushered in the era of metrics. Performance mattered and performance
was measured. Figures and statistics became pre-eminent, but only for things that
could be easily and readily measured. A positivistic paradigm prevailed in which
hard quantities and numbers forced out alternative, softer and less measurable, approaches to providing a service for citizens and communities. In the vernacular
of police officers, 'we did what could be counted, and not what couldn't be'. The
'Compstat' process, with its intense focus on statistics and holding officers to account, worked through in the New York Police Department under Mayor Giuliani
and Commissioner Brattan, was imported in varying degrees into the British policing system. And Chief Constables were held to account by government, and constables, and those in between were held to account, by their chief. Seduced by hard
data, politicians impressed accountability through performance and measures, and
created an instrumental and changed mindset in the police service.

At the same time, and through the 1990s, there emerged a public sector leadership development strategy. The strategy had, essentially, a singular focus: it directly
implied a relationship between organizational performance and effective leadership. The education service was the first to apply the policy. In 1998 the Department
of Education and Employment (DfEE) and Teacher Training Agency (TTA) commissioned Hay McBer, US based management consultants, to investigate the characteristics of highly effective headteachers and to construct a competency framework. The establishment of the National College for School Leadership in 2000
followed, and other public services proceeded to replicate the sectoral and organisational priority of leadership development. The National Policing Improvement
Agency (NPIA) was established by the Police and Justice Act 2006, with the remit
of 'the identification, development and promulgation of good practice in policing'

(Home Office 2012) in which, in the tradition of its predecessor Centrex (Central Police Training and Development Authority) which had established a Leadership Academy, leadership development was a key activity. By this time the orthodoxy and predominance of transformational leadership as the route to effective leadership was firmly embedded in its courses and publications, like the Core and Senior Leadership Development Programmes.

The Police Service was not alone in the course of action or the direction it took. The Fire and Rescue Service in England introduced a Centre for Leadership (CfL) with the purpose of improving leadership capability and capacity to effect modernisation and improve service delivery. By 2010 the National Health Service had a Leadership Academy and a Leadership Framework setting the standard for 'outstanding leadership at all levels and across all health professions' (http://www.nhs-leadershipqualities.nhs.uk/). The framework itself can be compared and contrasted with NPIA's own Police Leadership Qualities Framework (PLQF). The public services went hand in hand down the road of transformational leadership.

Arguably the two pronged approach, New Public Management and the public sector leadership development strategy, had a schizoid effect on the police service. It is reflective of what Savage (2007a) terms the bifurcation of police reform, a contradictory or paradoxical thrust, simultaneously, of empowerment and disempowerment. There was empowerment, on the one hand, of the 'street level' bureaucrats, with, for example, an emphasis on discretion, and the increasing role of the police officer in community engagement, representing this approach. Transformational imperatives and the notion that 'every officer is a leader', were part of this empowering strategy, but it was limited to an operational dimension. On the other hand, disempowerment applied at a strategic and policy level, as the police service lost control of its own destiny, insofar as it ever had it. The argument has received even greater force in recent years under the Coalition government, and what may be termed the Winsor reform agenda, on pay, conditions, and direct entry, and the removal of police authorities and their replacement by the direct election of PCCs holding Chief Constables personally to account.

At the heart of the leadership prescription was the drive towards transformational leadership as the prime mover of effective change. It was rooted within the heroic, industrial, leadership paradigm, built around visionary leadership, and, in terms of organisational crisis, the leader as saviour. Dobby et al. (2004) in their Home Office Report 'Police leadership: expectations and impact' established a very close link between effectiveness and the transformational approach: '53 specific behaviours were identified as being related to effective leadership, of which 50 were found to match closely with a style of leadership known as 'transformational'. Police leaders who displayed these 'transformational' behaviours were found, in the officers and staff questionnaire study, to have a wide range of positive effects on their subordinates' attitudes to their work, for example increasing their job satisfaction and their commitment to the organization' (pv). Transformational leadership was seen as key to leadership development in the police service.

Recent years have seen a challenge to this dominant orthodoxy, to the 'single most studied and debated idea within the field of leadership studies' since the 1980s

(Diaz-Saenz 2011, p. 299). It has been assaulted from both within and without the police service.

Van Knippenberg and Sitkin's (2013) forensic dissection of charismatic-transformational leadership research, and the 'imperial status' (p. 50) of the model, argues a lack of clarity in both conceptualising the leadership phenomenon and in operationalising it. Tourish (2013) has explored the psychological power dimensions, and thus the 'dark side of transformational leadership'. In the context of where the International Association of Chiefs of Police (1999) set out its stall, he cautions against reliance on the leader, where charisma can lead to narcissism. Further Alimo-Metcalfe and Alban-Metcalfe (2008) define much of the transformational perspective as being based upon 'distant leadership', that is, on empirical studies of CEOs and senior managers, research undertaken mostly in US with self-reporting white males who cast themselves in heroic roles and the leader as saviour, emphasising the importance of the chief executive and their charisma. Kellerman (2012) suggests there should be 'more emphasis on the role of followership as opposed to an infatuation with leadership' (p. 214).

Significantly, from within the police service, in his review of police leadership, Neyroud (2010) has contested the singular focus on transformational approaches, 'The main findings support the now common notion that transformational leadership has positive effects. However, studies suggest that the ability to apply different leadership styles, including transactional, to suit different contexts is the key to great police leadership' (p. 33). Additionally the report identified 'the relative lack of focus on front line leadership, whilst at the same time suggesting that attempts to introduce transformational leadership, to the exclusion of other more 'transactional' styles and behaviours, is neither appropriate nor likely to be effective' (p. 39).

What order of crisis, then, is the police service immersed in? Is it fundamentally a leadership crisis, deriving from 'distant' leaders who were required to drive performance and measurement rather than transform relationships between the police service and the community? Whatever its origins the focus on a leadership solution persists. In his report to the Home Secretary in March 2014, HM Chief Inspector of Constabulary, addressing the loss of public confidence, significantly, and perhaps all too predictably, added, 'It is primarily the responsibility of the leadership of the police to repair the damage which has been done' (para 8). But things might need to go beyond leadership. Interestingly Greiner's (1972, 1998) model which charts organisational growth in a business through evolutionary and revolutionary phases and crises, begins with a leadership crisis, early, in the foundation stage, and moves through crises of autonomy, control, and bureaucracy to an undefined and unpredictable crisis in its final stages. Can the police service reach beyond looking to some leadership strategy tailored to austere fiscal times to sustain a relationship with a public that is fast losing confidence in it?

If it is not a crisis, but an opportunity, then what is it an opportunity for? What then is the direction that the police service could take, assuming it can take control of its own direction as much as the centrally and locally democratic processes allow, and most of all, how can it re-affirm its Peelian roots, re-establish confidence amongst the public, and assure its legitimacy? Quo vadis?

Changing Directions

Lack of public confidence in the police is both symptom and cause of the current crisis, but HMIC has identified the relationship with the public as the key to cutting crime: "Neighbourhood policing is central to this, and it is from co-operation from the public at that level that the police obtain most of their information about crime and the potential for crime, whether it is in the roots of anti-social behaviour, leading to more serious crime, or for the purposes of counter-terrorism" (HMIC 2014b, p. 59). Further, listening to the views of local people and understanding the impact policing services has on communities is a key component of the National Police Vision 2016 (College of Policing 2014) and the Strategic Policing Requirement (Home Office 2015).This is part of a wider narrative however. Policing in its widest sense is being reconsidered at its political centre, and the 'language of change', explicit, for example, in Prime Minister Cameron's notion, of the 'Big Society', implies that communities will be expected to take on more social responsibilities, and work differently with the police in their areas (Stevens 2012). The question arising from this is how will the police interpret and deliver against this imperative, for this change of emphasis and direction comes at a time when public confidence in the police is diminishing and the police service is in a largely self-inflicted crisis? The problem therefore is how the police can engage with communities which are moving in the direction of disengagement.

Waters' (1996) model of 'quality service' in policing gives insight into how a new strategy of listening to citizens through a model of community engagement might be framed. Waters refers to three elements of the delivery of a quality service by the police: functional, internal quality, and interactional. The functional aspect embraces operational activity such as crime clear up rates and response times to emergency calls. The internal quality dimension is concerned with organisational culture, management and staff development. Interactional relates to inter agency partnerships, responding to community requirements and the provision of a reassuring police service. As the police struggle through repeated austerity driven transformational programmes, the functional and internal quality elements are given priority while the operational delivery of the interactional element remains the poor relation. Significantly, creating and building relationship through the interactional elements, might also be the key to restoring public confidence in the police.

Austerity has resulted in the police going through the tumult of restructure, resource reduction, new systems and new process. At the same time the focus remains firmly on performance relating to achieving targets (Metropolitan Police Federation 2014). In some cases the transformation programmes are in their second or third iteration as the police face the fourth consecutive year of real term reductions in government funding. While the focus is on these key issues, linking the internal quality and functional aspects of Waters' model, the interactional element, especially in relation to building relationships with communities, gets lost. As the government cuts bite deeper into police budgets the reduction in the workforce is becoming ever more apparent and this in turn leads to a risk to the efficacy of a decentralised neighbourhood policing function (Brain 2013; p. 219). The reduction in front line policing is acknowledged in the HMIC report Policing in Austerity: One Year On (HMIC 2012), but more concerning is the fact that the neighbourhood officer interactional role continues to be watered down by an increasing requirement to undertake response and investigative roles. This is a classic example of the interactional element of the Waters model being overtaken by the internal quality and functional elements.

Yet the logic of developing a structure that is capable of building interactional relationships with communities, increasing social capital, what Putnam (2000) defines as 'trust, norms and networks' that facilitate cooperation for mutual benefit, and using the assets that exist within communities to reduce crime is irresistible (Tyler and Fagan 2008). As Lord Stevens (2012; p. 57) writes, 'Public participation in police work has always been vital but it is becoming increasingly so: as police resources become ever tighter, utilising the 'hidden wealth' of social networks and voluntary activity in civil society to help contain and prevent crime is critical'. Further support for this position is provided by Myhill and Quinton (2011) who identify that positive public interaction is a key aspect of crime reduction as citizens tend to cooperate with the police. They go on to explain that, 'As this approach seeks to encourage people to become more cooperative and socially responsible on a voluntary basis, by "winning hearts and minds", it potentially offers a cost-effective way of reducing crime'. It is this cost effective solution that, in times of austerity, should be attracting the attention of police leaders as they battle to reduce crime on a reducing budget.

The opportunity of allowing the community constable to become the community leader as posited by Alderson (1998) and social diagnostician (Savage 2007b) is achievable; however, it requires the development of a new service model that moves away from a reliance on enforcement and chasing detections. As Myhill and Quinton (2011) state 'given that enhanced trust and legitimacy is likely to encourage voluntary public cooperation and would have a largely preventive effect on crime, a 'service' model of policing could help forces to avoid the financial costs resulting from an approach based narrowly on deterrence and punishment'. Police leadership is a key element that has to be addressed if this change in direction is to be achieved. Bringing community engagement into the realm of leadership and accountability, the Stevens report (2012; p. 18) argued that, 'The Commission believes that local community engagement has to be made a routine component of police work and a core responsibility of those elected to hold the police to account'. We often forget that policing by consent means that the police are held accountable by those whom they serve, the community, a fact commented upon by the Home Office (2010).

Police leadership in this instance does not only refer to those wearing stripes, pips, or crowns, where transformational strategies are generally espoused and focused, that is on the 'distant leader' (Alimo-Metcalfe and Alban-Metcalfe 2008), but to those who occupy the space with direct access to communities and who are able to influence citizens to take an increased role in policing their own communities. However, those wearing the insignia of rank must become enablers who understand the value of engaging communities and encourage front line officers to do so in a meaningful way. Active citizenship or social leadership is something that Alderson believed was a core function of the police mandate. Alderson (1979) was referring to the requirement that 'a future police system in a democratic society, can only be meaningful in the context of joint police community activity' (Alderson, 1979; p. 199). Alderson continued that he viewed the mobilisation of communities to achieve common goals as a key principle for the community officer as a community leader and that this person should 'provide leadership and participate in dispelling criminogenic social conditions through co-operative social action'. In other words the police and community need to work together to tackle the problem blighting communities, a clear reference to the trusts, norms and networks associated with social capital.

Increasing social capital and engaging communities can have a positive impact on levels of crime, trust and confidence in the police. MacDonald and Stokes (2006) found that depleted levels of perceived community social capital contribute to higher levels of distrust of local police and, similarly, Hawdon (2008) states that social capital influences resident perceptions of the police: the greater the levels of social capital, the greater the levels of trust. At a time when levels of trust and confidence are continually challenged as a result of the crises referred to earlier, there is a pressing requirement for the police to look to community engagement in order to redress the balance and start to build a new relationship with communities.

Successful police/community engagement relies on success in two areas. The first is the recognition that engaging communities requires an exact methodology. Selecting the right method or technique for the community is a crucial element. It involves research, data collection, coding and analysis. Reports proposing action or activities should be based on the findings and joint plans with the community and partner agencies should be developed. Community engagement involves criminological theories such as Broken Windows theory (Wilson and Kelling 1982), Problem Oriented Policing (Goldstein 1990), Informal Social Control (Carr 2003); it involves social science theories such as Social Capital (Putnam 2000) Social Contract (Rawls 1971) and theories relating to participation. An ability to understand and apply these theories goes some way to enabling the community officer, and we would now include PCSOs as they are a crucial element of community policing, to become the 'social diagnostician' referred to by Alderson (1998).

Community engagement needs police leaders and followers who understand this if they are to be prevented from 'reverting to type' and doing what they have always done, for example, holding sparsely attended police community forums, or relying on the posting of information flyers or surveys; in other words failing to change direction. This is at best community communication rather than community engagement as it fails to give citizens a voice or the opportunity for the police to listen. Achieving the 'interactional' element of the Waters model requires a style of leadership from senior officers that acknowledges the logic and power of building social capital in order to achieve the police mission to reduce crime. It requires leaders who are willing to do so by empowering front line officers, enabling them to develop their skills and removing the clutter of the functional and internal quality elements of performance targets.

This is no mean feat as the performance culture within the police, although mooted to be on its way out, is firmly rooted within the police service (Metropolitan Police Federation 2014). In relation to engaging communities this can mean counting the number of leaflets posted, the numbers of people attending events, the numbers of bikes protectively marked or the numbers of followers on social media sites. The command/control culture of police leadership poses many challenges for progressive leaders who genuinely want to empower the frontline to do the 'right thing', and who are open to iterative learning and reflection. It also poses many challenges for those on the front line who want to lead from the front and serve the community in a way that reflects their need. The reason for this is identified by Steinheider and Wuestewald (2008) who state that modern police organizations remain largely centralised in their decision-making, structurally vertical, rule bound, and mired in power relationships (Mastrofski 1998; Sklansky 2007). These limitations are seen as impediments to the development of adaptive, learning organizations capable of leveraging their human assets and appropriately responding to the dynamics of modern social expectations (Alarid 1999).

The search for a new direction and the willingness of police leaders to embrace new ideas and implement reform has been, in one global study, an interesting and commendable feature of the police profession (Das and Marenin 2009).

In its own reflection on lessons from the literature in relation to community engagement, the National Policing Improvement Agency (NPIA) identified that there was consistent theoretical evidence, based largely on the experiences of major programmes in the US, to suggest that strong leadership and effective management are essential to the implementation of community engagement (Myhill 2012). If this is the case it may well be that police leaders have to learn from acknowledged leaders in terms of service provision, and they may well have to look outside of the service for the expertise that exists in this area. The reason for this is identified by Bayley (1989) who elucidates that most innovations and reforms in the USA were not instigated by the police themselves but designed by people outside policing or generated by outside events and then offered to the police for adoption.

While the focus of police leadership training over recent years rests within the continuum of transactional—transformational styles with an emphasis on performance management, the change of direction posited here will likely require skills that exist outside of those models.

The test for police leadership is not only that it should value engaging communities, which has been a fundamental aspect of policing since the Peelian principles proclaimed, 'The police are the public and the public are the police', but whether it can make space for the training, facilitation and support that it requires for consistent provision rather than the reactive nature following crises such as the murder of Stephen Lawrence or the death of Mark Duggan. Perhaps the most obvious example of this is the fact that post the Duggan inquest result, the Metropolitan Police decided to appoint a senior officer to take charge of its community engagement, which prompted one police officer turned academic to ask what they have been doing for the last 185 years (Holdaway 2014).

Police leaders have to learn that community engagement is not an 18 month long project that sits neatly within the functional aspect of the Waters model, as an optional trial and error strategy. To be effective it has to involve a change of direction from a reliance on a hierarchical structure that is often cited as a major hindrance to front line officer empowerment, which community policing and problem-oriented policing (POP) seem to require (Goldstein 1990; Kelling and Coles 1996; Skogan 2004) to a participative style that brings together the major stakeholders in police organisations in collaborative decision making that offers promise for leader-follower relations, building employee commitment, improving public service, and reducing rank-and-file resistance to police reform initiatives (Skogan 2006; Steinheider and Wuestewald 2008).

Conclusion

The political imperative for the police from the Coalition government is clearly to reduce crime (May 2011). The drive for civil society with communities playing a greater part in directing public services and participating in joint action to solve their problems is also clear. The police have to deliver a reduction in crime against a background of reduced budgets, reduced resources and continual self-made crises that could result in a challenge to policing by consent. The case for building relationships with communities and increasing social capital is easily made, especially in times of austerity. Increasing social capital through community engagement is a new model for policing that could build levels of trust and confidence resulting in increased cooperation removing the necessity to rely on costly enforcement strategies. When viewed as a long term project, community engagement saves money. However, leadership and training are critical aspects. Training in the key methodological aspects of community engagement through a supported delivery process is essential. Leadership that empowers front line officers will enable them to identify and use the assets that exist within communities and develop joint problem solving strategies to increase the social welfare of citizens.

However, in order to decide so, senior leaders have to accept that they may have to look elsewhere for the expertise to do this and they then have to enable front line officers with the skills, support and time to develop long term relationships that are likely to pay dividends. It is appropriate to ask, whether, in this climate of crisis, the police service can afford not to. It is not just a matter of the police service putting its own house in order; there is a wider social responsibility resting on communities of sharing in the challenge of maintaining law and order. In this respect the police are nevertheless looked to, and well placed, to give the lead.

References

Adlam, R. (2002). Governmental rationalities in police leadership: An essay exploring some of the "Deep Structure" in police leadership praxis. *Policing and Society: An International Journal of Research and Policy, 12,* 15–36.

Alarid, L. F. (1999). Law enforcement departments as learning organizations: Argyris's theory as a framework for implementing community-oriented policing. *Police Quarterly, 2*(3), 321–337.

Alderson, J. C. (1979). *Policing freedom.* Plymouth: MacDonald and Evans.

Alderson, J. C. (1998). *Principled policing.* Winchester: Waterside Press.

Alimo-Metcalfe, B., & Alban-Metcalfe, J. (2008). *Engaging leadership: Creating organisations that maximise the potential of their people.* London: CIPD.

Bayley, D. (1989). Community policing in Australia: An appraisal. In D. Chappell & P. Wilson (Eds.), *Australian policing: Contemporary issues* (pp. 63–82). Sydney: Butterworths.

Boffey, D. (2014). Scotland Yard in new undercover police row. *The Observer.*

Bradford, B., Jackson, J., & Stanko, E. (2009). Contact and confidence: Revisiting the impact of public encounters with the police. *Policing and Society, 19,* 20–46.

Brain, T. (2013). *A future for policing in England and Wales.* Oxford: Oxford University Press.

Briggs, D. (2013). *The English riots of 2011: A summer of discontent.* Hook: Waterside Press.

Carr, P. J. (2003). The new parochialism: The implications of the beltway case for arguments concerning informal social control. *The American Journal of Sociology, 108*(6), 1249–1291.

Cohen, M. D., March, J. G., & Olsen, J. P. (1972). A garbage can model of organizational choice. *Administrative Science Quarterly, 17,* 1–25.

College of Policing. (2014). National policing position papers. https://www.app.college.police.uk/app-content/investigations/investigative-interviewing/national-policing-position-papers/. Accessed 29 April 2015.

Das, D. K., & Marenin, O. (2009). *Trends in policing: Interviews with leaders across the globe.* USA: CRC Press.

Diaz-Saenz, H. (2011). Transformational leadership. In A. Bryman, D. Collinson, K. Grint, & M. Uhl-Bien (Eds.), *The Sage handbook of leadership* (pp. 299–310). London: Sage.

Dobby, J., Anscombe, J., & Tuffin, J. (2004). *Police leadership: Expectations and impact, research development and statistics directorate.* London: Home Office.

Ferlie, E., Ashburner, L., Fitzgerald, L., & Pettigrew, A. (1996). *The new public management in action.* Oxford: OUP.

Ford, R. (2014). We regularly fiddle crime numbers, admit police. *The Times.*

Gargan, N. (2013). Police leaders must work hard to retain public confidence, Chief Constable argues. *Daily Telegraph.*

Golding, B., & Savage, S. (2008). Leadership and performance management. In T. Newburn (Ed.), *Handbook of policing* (pp. 725–759). Uffculme: Willan.

Goldstein, H. (1990). *Problem-oriented policing.* New York: McGraw-Hill.

Greiner, L. E. (1972). Evolution and revolution as organizations grow. *Harvard Business Review, 50,* 37–46.

Greiner, L. E. (1998). Evolution and revolution as organizations grow. *Harvard Business Review, 76,* 55–68.

Hawdon, J. (2008). Legitimacy, trust, social capital, and policing styles: A theoretical statement. *Police Quarterly, 11*(2), 182–201.

HMIC. (2012). *Policing in austerity: One year on.* London: HMIC.

HMIC. (2014a). *Everyone's business: Improving the police response to domestic abuse.* London: HMIC.

HMIC. (2014b). *State of policing: The annual assessment of policing in England and Wales 2012/13.* London: HMIC.

Holdaway, S. (2014). For how many years has it been recognised that community engagement is central to policing - 25+?. Now this http://tinyurl.com/o6hkqql http://tinyurl.com/o6hkqql #scc014. [Twitter]15 January. https://twitter.com/SimonHoldaway1/status/423391596499836929. Accessed 4 Sept 2014.

Home Office. (2010). *Policing in the 21st century: Reconnecting police and the people. Cm 7925*. London: Home Office.

Home Office. (2012). Home office framework document for: The National Policing Improvement Agency (NIPA).

Home Office. (2015). Strategic *policing requirement*. London: Home Office.

Hood, C. (1991). A public management for all seasons. *Public Administration, 69,* 3–19.

IACP. (1999). *Police leadership in the 21st century*: Recommendations from the president's first leadership conference: International association of chiefs of police. http://www.theiacp.org/Police-Leadership-in-the-21st-Century. Accessed 28 April 2015.

Kellerman, B. (2012). *The end of leadership*. New York: Harper Collins.

Kelling, G., & Coles, C. (1996). *Fixing broken windows: Restoring order and reducing crime in our communities*. New York: Touchstone. As cited in (Steinheider and Wuestewald 2008).

Loader, I. (2014). Police scandal and reform: Can we break out of more of the same? http://www.leftfootforward.org/2014/03/police-scandal-and-reform-can-we-break-out-of-more-of-the-same/. Accessed 4 April 2014.

MacDonald, J., & Stokes, R. J. (2006). Race, social capital and trust in the police. *Urban Affairs Review, 41,* 358–375. As cited in (Hawdon 2008).

Mastrofski, S. D. (1998). Community policing and police organizational structure. In J. Brodeur (Ed.), *How to recognize good policing: Problems and issues* (pp. 161–189). Thousand Oaks: Sage.

May, T. (2011). Police reform: Home secretary's speech on 2 March 2011 https://www.gov.uk/government/speeches/police-reform-home-secretarys-speech-on-2-march-2011. Accessed 28 April 2015.

Maybin, S. (2014). Do the public still trust the police? (WWW Document). BBC News Magazine. http://www.bbc.co.uk/news/magazine-26730705. Accessed 4 Jan 2014.

Metropolitan Police Federation. (2014). The consequences of a target-driven culture within policing: From the voices of metropolitan police officers. Metropolitan Police Federation.

Miller, P., & Rose, N. (1990). Governing economic life. *Economy and Society, 19,* 1, 1–31.

Myhill, A. (2012). *Community engagement in policing: Lessons from the literature*. Ryton: NPIA.

Myhill, A., & Quinton, P. (2011). It's a fair cop: Police legitimacy, public cooperation, and crime reduction an interpretative evidence commentary. National Policing Improvement Agency.

Neyroud, P. (2010). *Review of police leadership and training*. London: Home Office.

Normington, D. (2014). *Independent review of the police federation*. London: RSA.

Osborne, D., & Gaebler, T. (1992). *Reinventing government*. Reading: Addison-Wesley.

Putnam, R. D. (2000). *Bowling alone: The collapse and revival of American community*. New York: Simon and Schuster.

Rawls, J. (1971). *A theory of justice*. USA: Harvard University Press.

Reiner, R. (2010). *The politics of the police* (4th ed.). Oxford: OUP.

Sanders, A. (2013). "Policing in Gwent has a bad name": MP laments lack of applicants for chief constable vacancy (WWW Document). Wales Online. http://www.walesonline.co.uk/news/wales-news/policing-gwent-bad-name-mp-6189427. Accessed 4 Jan 2014.

Savage, S. (2007a). *Police reform: Forces for change*. Oxford: OUP.

Savage, S. (2007b). Give and take: The bifurcation of police reform in Britain. *Australian & New Zealand Journal of Criminology, 40,* 313–334.

Sklansky, D. (2007). Seeing blue: Police reform, occupational culture, and cognitive burn-in. In M. O'Neill & M. Marks (Eds.), *Police occupational culture: New debates and directions* (pp. 19–46). Oxford: Elsevier Science.

Skogan, W. G. (2004). Community policing: Common impediments to success. In L. Fridell (Ed.), *Community policing: The past, present, and future* (pp. 159–167). Washington, DC. Police Executive Research Forum. As cited in Steinheider, B., & Wuestewald, T. (2008). From the bottom-up: Sharing leadership in a police agency. *Police Practice and Research, 9*(2), 145–163.

Skogan, W. G. (2006). Why reforms fail. Paper for the University of Berkeley/Australian National University Conference on Police Reform from the Bottom-Up, Berkeley, CA. As cited in Steinheider, B., & Wuestewald, T. (2008). From the bottom-up: Sharing leadership in a police agency. *Police Practice and Research, 9*(2), 145–163.

Steinheider, B., & Wuestewald, T. (2008). From the bottom-up: Sharing leadership in a police agency. *Police Practice and Research, 9*(2), 145–163.
Stevens Lord. (2012). Policing for a Better Britain report of the Independent Police Commission.
Tourish, D. (2013). *The dark side of transformational leadership*. Hove: Routledge.
Tyler, T., & Fagan, J. (2008). Legitimacy and cooperation: Why do people help the police fight crime in their communities? *Ohio State Journal of Criminal Law, 6,* 231–275.
Van Knippenberg, D., & Sitkin, S. (2013). A critical assessment of charismatic—Transformational leadership research: Back to the drawing board? *The Academy of Management Annal, 7,* 1–60.
Waters, I. (1996). Quality of service: Politics or paradigm shift? In F. Leishman, B. Loveday, & S. P. Savage (Eds.), *Core issues in policing* (1st ed.) (pp. 205–217). Singapore: Longman Group.
Williams, C. A. (2003). Britain's police forces: Forever removed from democratic control? History & Policy, Policy Papers.
Wilson, J. Q., & Kelling, G. L. (1982). Broken windows: Police and neighborhood safety. *Atlantic Monthly, 249,* 29–38.
Winsor, T. (2011). The independent review of police officer and staff remuneration and conditions. Home Office.

Dr. Andrew C. Fisher is a former police superintendent who now works as an Associate Lecturer at Liverpool Hope University UK on the Police Leadership MSc programme. He is also the Director of Blue Locust Network Ltd, a consultancy specialising in police/community engagement and quality of service. Andrew writes and delivers training for the police in the Middle East and has had articles published in relation police leadership and the history and development of policing.

John M. Phillips is a Senior Lecturer in the Business School at Liverpool Hope University, UK. He is the Award Director for the MSc in Police Leadership, a programme developing the leadership capability of officers and staff in several police forces in the UK. He has written a number of journal articles on the concept of leadership and leadership education with particular application to the police service. He has also written several book chapters on culture and ethics.

Chapter 4
Initial Police Training and the Development of Police Occupational Culture

Julian Constable and Jonathan Smith

Introduction

This chapter is intended to extract, from the now voluminous literature on police occupational culture, ideas which could impact on the practice and policy concerning police culture and particularly initial police training. A research case study conducted recently by the first author on initial training in one police force in England will be used to provide empirical support for some of the issues raised.

Culture, Sub-Culture and Occupational Culture

The study of police occupational culture has its origins in a number of cross-cutting ideas. The first is the idea of *culture*, the study of which indicates that human social groups develop characteristics (language, dress, habits and artefacts) that delineate them from other groups and that these characteristics are communicated symbolically over time to new members (Tylor 1974). However, from this question by Tylor a number of further questions arise. These include; to what extent are cultural characteristics shared (and common to all societies) or distributed unequally and thus give rise to many, often opposed forms. In that sense, we may need to use the term

J. Constable (✉)
Anglia Ruskin University, Cambridge, UK
e-mail: Julian.Constable@anglia.ac.uk

J. Smith (✉)
Devon and Cornwall Police, Devon, UK
e-mail: jonathan.smith3@devonandcornwall.pnn.police.uk

© Springer International Publishing Switzerland 2015
P. Wankhade, D. Weir (eds.), *Police Services*, DOI 10.1007/978-3-319-16568-4_4

cultures rather than the singular, culture. How far cultures are accepted or resisted and to what extent are cultural forms considered to have positive or negative consequences and finally, can and should anything be done to change or manage these cultures?

The second is the idea that sub-cultures arise in which often deviant groups generate characteristics that demonstrate their difference from and opposition to a 'dominant culture.' These so-called 'sub-cultures' also perform the function of raising the status of their members both within and often without their confines (Cohen 1971). A number of questions arise here too. To what extent are sub-cultures different or similar to other, often dominant, cultures? Is their existence a positive or a negative phenomenon? Are sub-cultures largely internally generated or do they arise principally from external pressures that exist in societies and their associated economic, political and social characteristics? This also raises the question of the extent to which the agency of the person and of groups can change cultural beliefs and practices and in doing so generate multiple cultures. This point will be addressed more directly in relation to police occupational culture later in the chapter.

Thirdly, with respect to occupational culture, it has been demonstrated that in modern, industrialised societies one of the principle locations of individual and group identity is derived from work. The values, attitudes and behaviours associated with it are often shared with others and communicated over time in the workplace which gives rise to what is termed 'occupational culture' As Riesman (1955, pp. 177–178) argues, "The question of the meaning of work, of how it is experienced, is primarily a cultural problem; and cultures vary enormously in the way work is interpreted in their value-scheme." Furthermore, the study of deviant and 'dirty work' (Hughes 1958; Davis 1984) has demonstrated how some groups of workers have to adjust to potential social stigma. The key questions here are; to what extent are occupational cultures to be celebrated or derided and to what extent are they different to one another and to the dominant culture?

We find these questions and concerns reflected in the study of police occupational culture. Whilst it took some time for researchers to turn their attention to studying the police, when they did these were the kinds of questions and concerns that were reflected in the study of police occupational culture

Police Culture: Essential Features

Police culture has been studied now for well over half a century and we cannot possibly highlight all these issues connected to this in this brief chapter. We attempt only to highlight some key aspects that have been identified from this research and to raise some questions that we are left wrestling with from this.

Westley's (1953) pioneering study identified the effect of police work on the self-perception of officers whom, he found, often felt hostile to those they policed. Banton (1964) focussed on what was considered a well-functioning group, identified the discretionary nature of law enforcement and demonstrated the 'social' rather than legal or criminal nature of police work. This feature of police work was also supported by Bittner (2005). Skolnick (1966) highlighted the pre-occupation, for the police officer, with danger, authority and the need for efficiency. The concern with action, excitement, violence; the divisions created by an isolated and solidaristic community; the existence of authoritarian, conservative and suspicious sentiments are all thought to characterise the nature of police culture (Reiner 1992 cited in Waddington 1999). These studies portray a common set of thought processes and behaviours that apply to police work and contain a concern with their deleterious effects on the community as a whole, particularly in conflicted contexts. However, partly because the early studies had focused exclusively on uniformed, routine police work at the lowest level in the police organisation, the variation in police culture had not been well explored. Furthermore, there is a lack of connection in these early studies with the wider political context of policing which has more recently led to further developments in research on police culture.

This variation is well exemplified by a number of studies. Muir (1977) who identified that officers, even at the lowest level, differently negotiated the moral and intellectual challenges of 'street-level' policing. Other studies found the existence of antagonism felt by 'street cops' in relation to 'management cops' (Reuss-Ianni and Ianni 1983) and that officers engaged on mainly 'community' level work exhibited a softening in their approach to policing and a change in attitudes and skills (Miller 1999). Studies on gender and the police found differences between male and female officers and the existence of a 'macho' police culture that derided women officers (Heidensohn 1992). Some police cultures were considered to be very authoritarian or in some cases quite liberal (Fielding and Fielding 1991). Brodeur (1983) identified the existence of 'high' policing and 'low' policing. The former refers to what Brodeur sees as the policing of political activity that has come to dominate much of modern policing.' Low policing' refers to policing designed to deter people from criminality. Much of the existing literature concerns the latter but both forms of policing exhibit different cultural characteristics. Janet Chan's study on police in New South Wales, Australia argued persuasively that it was important to see police culture as plural and not singular, to acknowledge the agency of the officer in mediating influences on them and to allow for change as well as resistance in relation to cultural values and practices (Chan 1996, 1997). The studies above make strong connections with the politics of the police and express significant concerns with the deleterious effects of plural police cultures.

At the wider level, major inquiries into the police organisation in Britain have found significant problems with the cultural traits of police officers (principally their racist characteristics) that were considered to have had a profound impact on their capacity to engender the confidence and cooperation of the general population (Scarman 1981; Macpherson 1999). This has led to attempts to make changes to the behaviour and the attitudes of police officers through such schemes as Race Awareness Training and through programmes centred on the need to provide a 'good' standard of customer service. Moving away from the UK context for a moment, Chan (1996) identified the difficulties in changing police culture in the New South Wales Police when racism was identified as a key component of the culture of the police. One of the main problems in effecting change was the failure, according to Chan, to recognise the complexity of the relationship between structural change and the way in which police officers accommodate to it.

The negative aspects to police culture, sometimes referred to as the 'canteen culture,' feature strongly in other literature and although talk of a 'police culture' undoubtedly makes it appear more monolithic than it actually is, there are some common aspects frequently mentioned. Kirschman (2006), Holdaway (1989) and Fielding and Conroy (1994) highlight peer pressure, cynicism and resistance to change as important elements of this culture. Kleinig (1996) identifies police cynicism and HMIC (2003) highlight resistance to change, as did Young (1991, p. 151) who argues that this resistance:

> ... was so strong that changes in the police would only ever occur when irresistible and more powerful forces were brought to bear from outside, such as legislation or boards of enquiry. Much of this research was motivated by civil libertarian concerns about police malpractice and deviance.

Waddington (1999), however, considers many of the approaches to police culture (such as some of those above) as overly 'condemnatory' and argues that the value of academic research is to look beyond 'normative condemnation and to seek to appreciate (but not to condone) even the most offensive behaviour' (Waddington 1999, p. 294). The idea that Waddington conveys of the capacity of police officers to resist the stigmatising effects of those from the 'outside' by venerating what might be seen as 'dirty' work has a long tradition in social science (Hughes 1962). Waddington considers police culture to be singular and that studies that have stressed the variation in culture have, as a result, lost sight of its common characteristics and functions across all policing activities. Its enduring nature, despite a transitional period, has been supported by recent research by Loftus (2010). Waddington, goes on to argue that social scientists have tended to assume that what police officers say they do and the values they express (often in' off-guard' moments) are in fact translated into action. This he regards as erroneous and that, for the most part, the actions of police officers are motivated by situational variables such as the severity of an offence rather than malign intent caused by the application of pernicious occupational values. Furthermore, he argues that the strength of the occupational culture provides some protection from the potential stigmatising consequences of working as a police officer.

In this sense, the purpose of the 'chatter' of the canteen and other informal venues (which Waddington (op. cit) argues is the basis of the 'normative' and 'condemnatory' approach) is to give 'meaning to experience' and to ease the isolating experience of working as a police officer. So, when officers adopt a fatalistic attitude they do so as a means of coping with a fearful reality that might otherwise overwhelm them. For Waddington, there is a common police culture that transcends divisions (including race and gender) identified by some of the studies above but its features are not exclusive to the police or distinctive and defining characteristics. He writes that,

> Thus it is far from the case that the police are a repository for authoritarianism, racism and conservatism within a liberal population brimming over with the milk of human kindness.

Their sub-culture might be less 'sub' than is often supposed and instead be the expression of *common* values, beliefs and attitudes within a police context. (Waddington 1999, pp. 292–293)

An approach adopted and developed by Liebling et al. (2010), 'appreciative inquiry' applied in the context of the work of the prison officer allows an appreciation (rather than condemnation) of such cultural characteristics of 'gallows humour' that shares some similarities with the police and other emergency services. This perspective allows us to understand police culture without condoning its excesses and has informed the case study of police initial training detailed below. This may ameliorate the problem identified by Foster that the:

negative aspects [of police culture] have also been the predominant focus of academic research which leaves the police view of their own culture, and the academic research on it, in rather polarised positions. (Foster 2005, p. 199).

What follows is a discussion of the connections between some of the literature on police initial training and the issues of culture identified above.

Police Initial Training and Police Occupational Culture

The initial training environment is often seen as one of the most important and formative places where culture and particularly negative cultural traits originate. Hence the attempts to control and change the nature and content of initial training (HMIC 2002) with direct reference to the problems associated with cultural patterns (Scarman 1981). The historical examination of police initial training in England and Wales has seen frequent changes to initial training to take account of changes in the wider police policy environment and to rectify controversial problems identified at important junctures in the history of the police. Examples include changes following the inquiry by Lord Scarman into the Brixton riots in 1981 and the inquiry by Lord Macpherson in 1999, after the murder of Stephen Lawrence (Peacock 2010; Elliott et al. 2003). The more recent policy background to police initial training was given impetus by the HMIC report *Training Matters* (2002) which argued that it was no longer 'fit for purpose', being overly militaristic, insufficiently local and that 'probationers' were poorly supervised in the working environment. In this context, a new programme of initial training started in 2005 called the Initial Police Learning and Development Programme (IPLDP) that was intended to address the issues raised in *Training Matters* to make the programme more local and better tailored to the needs of officers in the work context. A report by the Adult Learning Inspectorate (2005) indicated that significant change had taken place, especially in relation to the community focus of the IPLDP. Here we would like to identify the key features of initial police training and the development of police occupational culture during this period of an officer's career. We will use examples from both the literature and the empirical material from the first author's case study of IPLDP. We hope to be able to demonstrate that the issues involved in the development of police

Table 4.1 Phases of initial police training

Phase one	Pre-patrol (Learning modules including OSTU)
Phase two	Consolidation (Tutored patrol)
Phase three	Independent patrol

culture during initial training clearly illustrate some of the key of police culture, raise some fundamental questions about police culture and the management of it, and that the study of police culture is complex and can be interpreted in a variety of ways.

The Case Study

A cohort of Student Officers (SOs) undertaking the IPLDP in a police force in England was selected on the basis of a study to understand the experience and the nature of the initial training programme and police culture. This training programme (see Table 4.1) commenced in June 2010 and finished in June 2012. The study followed a broadly qualitative approach using semi-structured interviews and observations. Interviews were carried out with 14 student officers at all stages in the programme and with constabulary staff managing this particular programme and those responsible for learning and development more generally in the force concerned. Observations of classroom learning, fitness testing and officer safety training were also undertaken. Field observations (where the researcher accompanied SOs on duty) were conducted during the longest period of initial training where officers worked as members of 'reactive' policing 'reliefs' in the force concerned. The study reflects an attempt to understand the issues concerned with initial training over the whole period of training and of the immediate period following it. The IPLDP studied, followed a format that demarcated between a number of pivotal progression points which allowed the SO and the force to understand individual development. These points also marked wider issues associated with the development of police culture although it is evident that those issues did not neatly fit the chronology of the programme.

Training as 'Groups'

One of the earliest studies of police initial training by Harris (1973) employed participant observation to study the early career training of American police officers and focussed specifically on the residential, pre-patrol phase. The issues addressed in Harris' study are remarkably similar to the concerns relating to police initial training currently and reflect the view that new recruits are not sufficiently exposed to 'liberal values'. Connected to this is the effect on officers starting their careers as part of military style squads which engenders a common cultural outlook. This has been very evident in the past (and police initial training has been criticised for it) in the UK context (HMIC 2002) and whilst it is a feature of the IPLDP, in this case study, it is also considerably different because of the absence of the erstwhile Central Training School. Student Officers in the study were trained in the force itself for the entire duration of the IPLDP. The groups that were formed reflected the divisions in existence in the force as a whole and their manifestations in the intra-force Basic Command Units (BCUs). The kinds of 'squad' described by researchers such as Harris (1973) and van Maanen (1971) and exemplified by activities like drill and neo-located, barrack style residence did not exist in the case study. There was no 'academy' or 'residential' phase in the IPLDP in this force but SOs did move from Induction to what were called Police Development Units (PDUs) where the initial larger group was disaggregated to the BCU located units. This gave rise to some interesting variations in approaches to training which is discussed below). SOs experience of the Learning Modules (LM) phase or the 'classroom' phase, as it was often called, reflected the attachment that SOs felt toward the particular pedagogy and staff of the PDU. Police law was the main focus for classroom work but the atmosphere in the PDU was set from the beginning. In one division this mirrored the Central Training School approach of the past (Peacock 2010) and extra emphasis was placed on rote learning of legal definitions and standards of behaviour and dress—precisely the approach so heavily criticised by HMIC (2002). The manager of that PDU felt under-pressure to defend the approach to colleagues and was well aware that other PDUs took a more flexible approach. One SO described it in this way:

> Our shirts have got to have one crease in the sleeve, on each sleeve, creases down the back of the shirt. Can't think what you call it at the top of the shirt. The Sergeant likes the crease straight down the centre, right the way from the top of the shirt to the bottom of the shirt. Trousers to have a sharp crease in them. Be clean and tidy and the boots to be clean but the tips of the boots to be 'bulled' almost like a parade 'bull'. So, we do that on a regular basis. We've had uniform inspections. We've had pocket notebook inspections. We've had feedback on our notes we've put that in our pocket notebooks.

Another PDU had a reputation for a little eccentricity but where strong personal bonds were created with SOs. The Trainer there expressed a pedagogical approach that stressed the need to blend 'classroom' learning and 'practical' learning. In the remaining PDU the atmosphere was considered relaxed and a little' motherly.' This partially reflected the divisional cultural differences long existent in the force. SOs indicated that they had heard more experienced officers say that it felt like there were three different forces rather than one unified one. SOs tended to defend the approach taken by their division but officers from the 'stricter' division saw their time as harder than the other divisions, a situation they were proud of. They felt that this made them better SOs. An SO from one of the other PDUs did though hanker after the more formalised and militaristic approach and decried what she saw as an over-concerned approach taken by the trainers and managers of her PDU.

Motivation

Fielding's (1988) study of police training indicates that officers in that study joined for altruistic reasons but quickly became defensive in their outlook. One of the SOs in the case study, who was searching for a direction in life after pursuing a career that she had lost motivation for said that she decided to apply (to the police) because she wanted to 'help people.

> It's the massive cliché…something I'd always thought I wanted to do…I felt that being part of the police, it was helping people, it was varied work, it was challenging, you were doing something good for the community and it seemed to be quite well paid, so it seemed like a really interesting job to do.

However, the cohort in this study was constituted only in part of SOs completely new to policing. Many had served as PCSOs, Special Constables and Police Staff and their sense of altruism from the beginning was consequently much less visible than that of the SOs new to the process.

The Development of Cultural Characteristics

The idea that the new recruit to the police engages in the acquisition of its culture and is not just a recipient of its imposition is a key feature of some studies of initial training. Fielding (op. cit, p. 9) writes that,

> Consequently, the formal/informal model of socialisation into occupations remains only partial unless account is taken of the mediation of these influences by individuals making their own adaptations, constructing an 'organisational reality' special to themselves from these various sources of influence. The research data reveals the resilience of recruits and their capacity to resist as well as embrace the influences arising from formal and informal sources.

A study of 'probationer' officers in Britain by Fielding (1988) found that they were inducted into a pre-existing but complex occupational context and they contribute to its regeneration and to its transformation as they develop as police officers. These officers were seen to be actively selecting the aspects of the differentiated culture that they found acceptable. In the case study, it was very noticeable that SOs differentiated between one another, as did their training staff differentiate between them. One particular officer displayed a liberal, relaxed but also confident approach to policing that did not endear him to some of his peers. He was though considered sufficiently competent to progress very quickly to the Independent phase. He considered this a compliment but felt abandoned to the 'hustle and bustle' of 'reactive' policing. Other officers considered some of their peers somewhat 'loose cannons', overly aggressive. Some SOs experienced significant alterations in their personal lives and relationships developed between SOs on the programme and between SOs and longer serving officers that were partly a product of the intensity of the SOs working environment and the enormous changes they were undergoing.

The Police Bureaucracy

The way in which the new recruit experiences the police bureaucracy is an important element of Harris' (1973) study and he argues that it is experienced in a defensive way. As he writes,

> To the recruit, the rules seemed to indicate that he was essentially distrusted by the public and, perhaps, even by his own department…the rules and procedures intended to protect the officer were perceived by the recruit as another body of rules from which he would have to protect himself in the course of his duties. (Harris 1973, p. 33)

SOs in the case study experienced the process of application and recruitment as a bureaucratic one and not one designed to allow the force to understand them as individuals. The application process followed national standardisation criteria, took some considerable time to complete and often appeared to the prospective SO as both too easy and too formalised. Furthermore, as part of the IPLDP in the force in the study SOs completed a programme called Putting People First (PPF) which formed a part of the induction period for all SOs and was often experienced as problematic for them. The programme met with some scepticism from some SOs and the inherent dilemma in this programme (which was tacitly understood and occasionally verbalised) was described very well by a SO who said,

> PPF is good to an extent but it depends who you've got and how they're being with you. If somebody is being nice…and even if they're being horrible, you'll try and put them first but if they're being that bad, it's like well hang on a minute I'm a person as well. I'll put me first and I'm still putting somebody first. I'll put me first and I'll look after myself first before I'll help you. If you're gonna be like that with me and be nasty to me and shirty with me, I won't try and help ya…They didn't really discuss the idea that some people are difficult to put first…It just seemed like, you put everybody first and it's only really now, speaking with your PDO, "yeah, you put everybody first, when you can." In induction it just felt it couldn't be challenged.

There was, though, evidence of attempts made by training officers, senior operational officers and other parts of the training bureaucracy to facilitate a variety of problems that SOs had in completing their training that indicated that the bureaucracy was flexible rather than rigid. Extra role-plays, 1:1 meetings and extended time limits were not uncommon to allow SOs to complete their programme and as such some SOs came to see the force bureaucracy as supportive of their needs.

Teaching, Learning and Education

Harris (*op cit* 1973) argues that new recruits received an essentially vocational education despite the existence and acceptance of higher education qualifications in policing in the US context where police students were thought of as outsiders. In this sense, Harris (1973) argues that new recruits were not exposed during the 'Academy' phase, to a variety of ways of understanding the police role (especially liberal ones). In the UK context attempts have been made to unite the police and higher education worlds but these have not been systematic and have encountered a number of problems, not least of all, concerning a clash of the police and academic cultures (Wood and Tong 2009). Foster (1999) argues that if new recruits were to be required to have higher education qualifications upon entry they would be more likely to demonstrate more 'tolerant' and 'reflective' operational skills. Of the SOs in the case study, 3 had prior higher education experience in a range of subject areas. One SO with a degree in law certainly reflected the kind of 'tolerant' officer Foster (1999) describes and had a 'hard time' accommodating to the less tolerant approaches of his peers and colleagues. The other two in the cohort displayed much less conflicted approaches to police training and its environment and other factors were as important, in influencing their approaches to policing concerning gender, age and family background.

Stanislas (2012) on the other hand is one of those critical of the kind of instrumental approach to learning amongst students in higher education in general and particularly of the poor academic work of students on policing programmes in higher education.

The paucity of the 'competence based education and training' in existence in police initial training is thought by Hyland (1994) and Norris (1991) to fail to capture the process of learning, foster critical reflection or to address alternative perspectives. In the case study SOs progressed to the stage known as 'Independent,' after approximately 36 weeks of the programme. This was also the stage where SOs were required to complete an electronic portfolio of their learning and development known as the E-SOLAP. This was commonly and openly denigrated by SOs and those involved in managing it alike and its completion was encouraged to be as perfunctory as possible. "Don't do more than is required mate!' is how one supervisory officer advised SOs concerning its completion. One of the latter recognised the perception of the portfolio by himself using the epithet known by many undertaking it, the 'e-So crap!' Cutting and pasting of material from often poorly sourced online information, used to support the demonstration of the completion of occupational competences, was acknowledged without censor as a common practice. That the E-SOLAP needed to be completed as a condition of Confirmation was though held over the heads of SOs as a legal requirement and that it was subject to 'reg13', a reference to the Police Regulations that govern police conditions of service and facilitate the swift removal of SOs from the force at any point prior to Confirmation should they contravene it.

The 'Independent' phase was by far the longest period (72 out of 104 weeks) and contained a number of points of crisis and success that came to define SOs development as police officers. For example, for some SOs it marked the point at which they felt the need and necessity to distance themselves from the past and from those outside the police world. For one SO, there was a point which he described as an 'epiphany' where he came to realise the importance of equanimity and dialogue in policing but conversely its absence in the behaviour of other officers. This contradiction proved to be the eventual cause of his departure from the programme.

For some authors, police training has tended toward rigid forms of teaching by rote (Oliva and Compton 2009), has been fixated on law (to the detriment of other features of policing) and has failed to engage the active participation of new recruits (White 2006). This leads to a fear that SOs are able to act and think only in linear and legalistic ways. This was a feature of the Learning Modules phase for some of the recruits on the programme in the case study, especially in the BCU with a reputation for a disciplinarian approach. However, other BCUs had a more flexible, investigatory approach to learning with more time for exploration and individual research. The use of role-play as a teaching and learning tool was common until Independence. It was not always experienced favourably by SOs who thought it so artificial and removed from the operational environment as to be unhelpful to them. One SO, describing the whole experience of role-play said,

> Ok. An example would be in one of the role-plays you had to breathalyse someone. But in the role-play you know the person was a police officer…and the difference between that and a member of the public you want to breathalyse is immense. You're not stood in a nice safe yard in daylight with no one walking past. You're stood at the side of the road with the cars whizzing past you…You know what this is going to show. You're remembering bits of what you've been told. Hold on to the machine so they can't pull it off you. Hold it so they can't see the number. But it's completely different breathalysing a real member of the public…There are some things, I'm glad I did that role-play but it doesn't prepare you for the reality of going out and doing the job.

In the mind of the SO role play was sometimes experienced as a device to 'trip them up' and not an activity that fosters an exploratory approach to the development of skills. Nevertheless, feedback to the officer at an individual level was frequently given and some SOs struggling with the whole idea of performing in front of an audience received considerable extra help.

Danger and Authority

A concern in the literature on police culture (as noted above) was the over-focus on danger and authority to the detriment of a more expansive 'social service' understanding of the role of the police officer. This was well exemplified, in the case study, when all SOs took part in and completed a two week Officer Safety Training programme during the Learning Modules phase (classroom based) at the Officer Safety Training Unit (OSTU). This unit was a former military base where the principle training room was designed in the style of a karate dojo. This phase was of concern to some SOs, especially those that had no prior policing experience, because of their fears about their capacity to use force, which was played upon by trainers who occasionally took perverse pleasure in observing officers struggle with the holds and restraints practiced and with the idea of using force against another person. The pedagogical approach centred upon demonstration and role-play. The latter stages of the OSTU course was thought by one SO to be a much more 'real' context for role-play where they ended one particular activity on the floor attempting to restrain another role-play character. SOs were acutely aware they would be required to perform the summative, terminal assessment to the satisfaction of the trainers and that this was a point of the training that could 'make or break' them. Nevertheless, on occasions SOs displayed what trainers considered inappropriate delight in using restraints and such personal protective equipment as batons and sprays. This behaviour was swiftly and forcefully terminated in the case of one SO who was un-ceremoniously removed from an activity after being heard to say to a suspect whom he felt needed to be 'sprayed' to effect an arrest, "You're goin down buddy." Trainers also, contrary to their somewhat para-militaristic appearance, were willing to help bolster less confident and competent SOs in their completion of the tasks necessary for successful completion of the programme. This was particularly the case for some of the female SOs who experienced difficulties with the physical aspect of the safety training programme.

Initial Police Training and Culture

The discussion of police culture earlier indicated a contested terrain where researchers had reached often opposed conclusions about police occupational culture that stressed variously its complexity or its homogeneity and its need to be condemned or appreciated. The results from the case study fieldwork highlighted a number of features of initial training as was practiced in the force concerned which drew recruits, often unconsciously, into a police culture. Firstly, the shortcomings of competence based education and training are evident in the low status of the assessment process and especially the submission of evidence of occupational competence tended to reinforce a feature of police culture as anti-academic. Secondly, the nature of the hidden/uncodified and restrictive (often not so hidden) culture is evident in all phases of the training observed, especially in relation to dress, behaviour and curriculum content. However, this was fragmented in the force concerned and experienced differently depending on the more or less flexible approach to learning, highlighting the sub-cultural aspects discussed earlier Thirdly, there were many opportunities that were lost, especially at the start of the programme, where time was available for a more expansive and reflective initial period of training that addressed the wider role of the police. This reinforced the cultural preoccupation of the police in its task orientation and its pragmatism. The responses of the force to the changes in police training indicate a somewhat conservative approach perhaps shaping a risk averse, resistant to change culture lacking innovation

As student officers moved into the independent period of training problems connected with support for individual development, pressures of reactive policing, inconsistencies of operational practice between reliefs and the low status of particular elements of assessment have all emerged. However, it is also evident that the force in question has made attempts to support and to facilitate a variety of approaches to policing expressed and exemplified by some of the SOs in the study.

Conclusion

The exploration, so far, of culture and initial police training raises two fundamental questions. Firstly, is police culture shaped by internal, police factors or external ones derived from wider society and prior personal experience? The answer to this question has significant implications for the issue of whether police culture can be changed and managed within the police, or is it that a larger societal change is required if any cultural change in the police is to be seen.

Secondly, does the nature of police work, and particularly the 'dirty work,' shape officers behaviour, so that behaviours are developed and taught which are essential in order for police officers to cope with their work, or is the police culture developed for some other reason? This has major implications for any cultural change programmes in the police. If the police culture is developed, or is a demonstration of a coping mechanism for the dirty work then cultural change programmes which seek to change the police culture may well be doing a major disservice to police officers and ultimately to those members of the public they serve.

The study of initial police training is an ideal focus and is ideally placed to help address some of these questions. The findings from the empirical study by the first author indicate that some of the features of police occupational culture, so well identified in the classic studies, remain in place and are nascent during initial training. SOs exhibit sentiments that demonstrate the development of a defensive attitude to others outside the police service, feel beleaguered by bureaucracy (especially one that stresses quality of service for all), dwell upon and are excited by the possibility of danger, work hard to at least appear to be in authority in operational situations and their approach to learning is pragmatic rather than developmental and often anti-academic. These features arise in both the officers' prior orientation to the police and in the course of training and would certainly incline us toward the view that the police themselves must not be the only party in cultural change programmes for the service.

However, other cultural features were not present or were seen in a different form to those suggested by some earlier studies. For example, there was no training in the kinds of large, residential (for a part of training) groups, that was a feature of initial training in some studies (Harris 1973; Fielding 1988). Consequently, SOs bonded with one another in relation to their respective Divisions rather than just as SOs. Indeed some considerable tension was noted as one of the PDU managers implemented a militaristic approach redolent of the old Central Training Schools. This clashed with the evidently more liberal approach at other PDUs. The pre-existing cultures (city vs rural and urban vs cosmopolitan) in the force as a whole were as powerful influences for the SOs as a general pressure to conform to the police culture identified in the literature. Furthermore, some SOs expressed sentiments and said that they took certain actions as police officers that seemed evidently to reject the approaches of their more authoritarian colleagues. It would seem that the work itself can generate a variety of cultural reactions to it and that some should be enhanced and others diminished. The work though takes place in an organisational context that is itself located in the prevailing social, political and economic context. Attempts to change one without reference to the other could be futile. Moreover, some of the occupational characteristics of the police, developed and nurtured during initial training, are necessary tools for all police officers to have to inure them from the difficulties they face in their work.

There might be a case for considering specific changes to initial policing training. Some elements of 'input' are seen to be so far removed as to be of little value to the SO. This might free up some time for more expansive learning activities. Role-play might be embedded better into the formative and summative assessment activities. They are experienced by some SOs as being too distant from operations and too unrealistic to be of significant benefit in their progress. In the periods where SOs were asked to conduct group work, the activities and materials might have been better directed at *bona fide* academic, policy and operational materials. Embedding safety training for SOs into the programme as a whole would be quite useful. This was almost entirely experienced as highly useful training for confidence building but as too removed from its real implementation. Further engagement should be sought, in relation to initial training, with HE but with a view to a form of collaboration that allows the best practices from both organisations to be used.

References

Adult Learning Inspectorate. (2005). *Evaluation of the New Initial Police Learning and Development Programme.* S.l.

Banton, M. (1964). *The policeman in the community.* Ney York: Basic Books.

Bittner, E. (2005). Florence Nightingale in search of Willie Sutton. In T. Newburn (Ed.), *Policing. Key readings.* Cullompton: Willan.

Brodeur, J. P. (1983). High policing and low policing: Remarks about the policing of political activities. *Journal of Social Problems, 30*(5), 507–520.

Chan, J. B. L. (1996). Changing police culture. *British Journal of Criminology, 36*(1), 109–134.

Chan, J. B. L. (1997). Changing police culture: Policing in a Multicultural Society. Cambridge: Cambridge University Press.

Cohen. (1971). Delinquent Boys: *The Culture of the Gang.* New York: New York Free Press.

Davis, D. (1984). Good people doing dirty work: A study of social isolation. *Symbolic Interaction, 7*(2), 233–247.

Elliott, J., Kushner, S., Alexander, A., Danes, J. D., Wilkinson, S., & Zamarski, B. (2003). *Independent review of the learning requirement for police probationer training. The learning, training and organisational requirements and the evidence base.* Home Office: London.

Fielding, N. G. (1988). *Joining forces: Police training, socialisation and occupational competence.* London: Routledge

Fielding, N., & Fielding, J. (1991). Police attitudes to crime and punishment: certainties and dilemmas. *British Journal of Criminology, 31* (1), 39–53.

Fielding, N., & Conroy, S. (1994). Interviewing child victims: police and social work investigations of child sexual abuse. *Sociology, 26* (1), 103–124.

Foster, J. (1999). "Appendix 22: Memorandum by Dr Janet Foster, Institute of Criminology, University of Cambridge". In *Home Affairs Committee, Police Training and Recruitment: Volume Two.* London: The Stationery Office, pp. 382–391.

Foster, J. (2005). Police cultures. In T. Newburn (Ed.), *Handbook of policing.* Cullompton: Willan.

Harris, R. N. (1973). *The police academy: An inside view.* New York: Wiley.

Heidensohn, F. (1992). *Women in control?* Oxford: Clarendon Press.

Her Majesty's Inspectorate of Constabulary. (2002). *Training matters.* London: Home Office Communications Directorate.

Her Majesty's Inspectorate of Constabularies. (2003). Diversity Matters. http://www.justiceinspectorates.gov.uk/hmic/media/diversity-matters-full-report-20030201.pdf. Accessed 1 April 2015.

Holdaway, S. (1989). Discovering structure: Studies of the British Police Occupational Culture. In M. Weatheritt (Ed.), Police Research: Some Future Prospects. Aldershot: Avebury.

Hughes, E. (1962). Good people and 'dirty work.' *Social problems, 10* (1), 3–11.

Hughes, E. (1958). Men and their work. London: The Free Press of Glencoe. https://archive.org/details/mentheirwork00hugh. Accessed 1 April 2015.

Hyland, T. (1994). *Competence, education and NVQs.* London: Cassell.

Kleinig, J. (1996). *The ethics of policing.* Cambridge: Cambridge University Press.

Kirschman, E. (2006). *I love a cop: what police families need to know.* New York: Guilford Publications.

Liebling, A., Price, D., & Shefer, G. (2010). *The prison officer.* Cullompton: Willan.

Loftus, B. (2010). Police occupational culture: Classic themes altered times. *Policing and Society, 20*(1), 1–20

Macpherson, Sir W., (1999). *The Stephen Lawrence Inquiry: Report of an inquiry by Sir William Macpherson of Cluny. (Cmnd 4262–1).* London: HMSO.

Miller, S. L. (1999). *Gender and community policing: Walking the talk.* Boston: North Eastern University Press.

Muir, W. K., Jr. (1977). *Police: Streetcorner politicians.* Chicago: UCP.

Norris, N. (1991). The trouble with competence. *Cambridge Journal of Education, 21*(3), 331–341.

Oliva, J. R., & Compton, M. T. (2009). What do police officers value in the classroom? *Policing: An International Journal of Police Strategies and Management, 33*(2), 321–338.

Peacock, S. M., (2010). *Initial Police Training in England and Wales.* EdD. University of East Anglia. https://ueaeprints.uea.ac.uk/10595/1/Thesis_peacock_s_2010.pdf. Accessed 18 Sept 2014.

Reiner, R. (1992). The politics of the police. 2nd edn. London: Wheatsheaf.

Riesman. (1955). *Individualism Reconsidered.* New York: Anchor Books.

Reuss-Ianni, E., & Ianni, F. (1983). Street cops and management cops: the cultures of policing. In M. Punch (Ed.), *Control in the police organisation.* Cambridge: MIT Press.

Scarman, L. (1981). *The Scarman report: The Brixton disorders. (Cmnd 8427).* London: HMSO.

Skolnick, J. (1966). *Justice without trial.* New York: Wiley.

Stanislas, P. (2012). *Extending civilisation: Challenges and dilemmas facing University-Based Police Education in Britain.* S.n.

Tylor, E. B. (1974). *Primitive culture: Researches into the development of mythology, philosophy, religion, art, and custom.* New York: Gordon Press.

Van Maanen, J. (1973). Observations on the making of policemen. *Human Organisation, 32*(4), 407–418.

Waddington, P. A .J. (1999). Police (canteen) sub-culture: An appreciation. *British Journal of Criminology, 39*(2), 287–309.

Westley, W. A. (1953). Violence and the police. *American Journal of Sociology, 59* (1), 34–41.

White, D. (2006). A conceptual analysis of the hidden curriculum of police training in England and Wales. *Policing and Society, 16*(4), 386–404.

Wood, D., & Tong, S. (2009). The future of initial police training: a university perspective. *International Journal of Police Science and Management, 11*(3), 294–305.

Young, M. (1991). *An inside job: Policing and police culture in Britain.* Oxford: Oxford University Press.

Julian Constable is Senior Lecturer in Public Services at Anglia Ruskin University and started his occupational life in the Police Service. He has been focusing on initial police training for his MPhil/PhD. His research is part evaluation, part sociological research on the new Initial Police Learning and Development Programme (IPLDP). He is interested in the teaching and learning strategies and methods used by students and trainers in the police service. The research also concentrates on understanding better the kind of police officer that emerges from initial training produces.

Dr Jonathan Smith, Chartered FCIPD is the Leadership Development Manager at Devon and Cornwall Police. Prior to this he was a Senior Lecturer at the Lord Ashcroft International Business School at Anglia Ruskin University, and prior to this a Director of Studies at the NPIA. He is a Fellow of the Leadership Trust, Member of the International Academic Advisory Board on Leadership in FE, Associate of the Centre for Governance, Leadership and Global Responsibility at Leeds Metropolitan University, Director of the Institute for Spirituality in Policing, and Member of the CIPD's Membership and Professional Development Committee. Co-author of many journal articles and books on leadership and policing including MisLeadership (2010), Ethics in Human Resource Management (2013), Developing Leadership Resilience: Lessons from the Policing Frontline (2013) and his latest book Co-Charismatic Leadership: Critical Perspectives on Spirituality, Ethics and Leadership (2014).

Chapter 5
Community Engagement, Democracy and Public Policy: A Practitioner Perspective

Susan Ritchie

Introduction: The Personal is Political

It's a phrase strongly associated with second wave feminism, but I explore it here to highlight the need for a better understanding of the personal if democracy is to survive and flourish in the UK. Bringing the personal and the political together could strengthen civic society, improve social policy, and reconnect the personal experiences of 'the people' with the political machinery of democratic governance, specifically the unelected arms of the state: police, local authorities and the National Health Service (NHS). Democratic engagement based on better ways of understanding the personal could help build new social norms, improve trust and dialogue, and create new social policy and public services which genuinely help the vulnerable.

This chapter outlines a personal experience of learning about democracy and considers why better forms of dialogue are essential if the public is to be served well politically. In the first half I outline my personal journey into *thinking* about democracy, and in the second half my experiences of *acting* to improve our democracy. I use both to call on my peers to help us all think and act in a way that could change the practice of Police and Crime Commissioners (PCCs), the (unelected) police and wider public sector officials, and just as importantly the general public.

S. Ritchie (✉)
MutualGain, 10 Tenby Road, RM6 6NB Essex, UK
e-mail: susan@mutualgain.org

© Springer International Publishing Switzerland 2015
P. Wankhade, D. Weir (eds.), *Police Services,* DOI 10.1007/978-3-319-16568-4_5

The Catalyst

I was a 19-year-old 'disengaged' citizen ignorant of the power of politics on my life, and the 'social' policy that emerges from political[1] decision-making. Unmarried and faced with teenage pregnancy, I quickly learned about social housing policy: Prime Minister Thatcher's 'Right to Buy' scheme was well under way and we were experiencing a gap in supply and demand of social housing (council housing was being offered to tenants to buy at a significantly reduced rate). The strict eligibility criteria to access a social housing property did not apply to me so my only option was to buy or rent privately.

Forced to move out of London and buy somewhere 'affordable', I quickly learned about monetary and fiscal policy: the mortgage was easy to secure, but within a matter of a few months the mortgage payments had more than doubled due to increased mortgage interest rates. Rather than 'fail', I rented the house out and went back to live with my dad, heavily pregnant with my second child. I hoped that if my partner and I rented the house out for 6 months we could move back in when the mortgage rates reduced again.

After receiving a letter from the mortgage company explaining that we didn't have permission to rent and neither did we have the right mortgage for renting, the bank took action and repossessed our house. The tenant had informed them of our apparently 'illegal' activity and was allowed to remain in our house whilst we faced in excess of £20k negative equity and no home. At 20 years old, I couldn't understand what I had done wrong.

Homeless with two children under 2 years old, we worked all hours to make ends meet so that we could create a home for our children. We weren't entitled to benefits because we were working (and no minimum wage then!). I would not have considered going to my MP nor would I have participated in any public meetings—I was busy trying to survive. Times were tough—I remember my mum giving me £5 and it was £5 I hadn't budgeted for. Should I spend this on nappies, food or some beer! Of course the beer didn't win, but the point is that £5 seemed a huge amount of unexpected money. If there were food banks then we would probably have used one.

Some months later my life took a turn for the better. It was near to the day of the repossession, and I was desperate for help. I walked into an insurance company thinking that they might be able to help me because they deal with money (ignorance is not always bliss!). There a wonderful stranger took pity on me when I asked for help and he changed the direction of my life, for which I will be eternally grateful. He took me in a room and gave me some advice which he made me promise never to tell anyone in any authority. Then he gave me a fatherly lecture and I went on my way to put his advice into action. We were back on the property ladder in a pretty dismal 'home' but we had a new start.

Determined to avoid such awful circumstances again I knew I needed a job which paid more money. That made me think about education policy: a change in

---

[1] I use the word political in the loosest sense of the word: it refers to the small 'p' politics played out in police forces, councils, and national health services on a daily basis, and the large 'P' politics of politicians who represent us.

school admissions policy meant I didn't go the grammar school as planned, and instead went to the school which had places, and as any parent will know, the school which has places usually has challenges. It would now be considered a 'failing school'; in fact it was shut down the year after I left. I had a lot of fun at school but managed to go through 5 years of secondary school education without doing a page of homework! I had a series of temporary 'teachers' who sat at the front of the class whilst we were disruptive. At 15, I left because there seemed no point in staying, and no one informed my parents or questioned my decision.

With no qualifications I knew I needed to go back to school. Juggling work with children I returned to college to do a computer course to develop my office skills. That was a good move; it secured me a job as a receptionist in a bank (better pay and conditions than the cab offices and waitressing jobs). I only discovered recently that the Computer Literacy and Information Technology (CLAIT) course which I completed was specifically designed for learners who were from 'deprived' and 'disadvantaged' backgrounds—more social policy which impacted upon my life.

As polytechnics converted to universities, and colleges extended their offer to meet a new 'market', access courses were being offered everywhere. They were a great opportunity for people like me, so a year after the CLAIT course, I registered on an Access to Higher Education course. My formal introduction to 'democracy' had started. Our six-week block of politics inspired me: it made sense to me but made me thirsty for more knowledge: social class, electoral systems, political parties and homelessness were four of the topics that challenged my thinking. My big questions were: *"why doesn't anyone teach you about politics in school? and why don't policy makers seek the views of those they are supposedly 'serving'?"* That has driven my career since, first developing my thinking about democracy and then trying to put some ideas into practice. I still think politics should be taught in schools but I am less convinced that teachers are the best people to teach it, unless they are well supported to do so. The same applies to public servants in policing, health, and councils—they aren't always well placed to know what is 'best' for those they serve, and should therefore be supported to develop better forms of dialogue with them.

By unlocking the experiences of the public and their resources we have an opportunity to refresh our democracy and build social capital in some of our most deprived areas with some of our most disadvantaged communities. *We have no choice but to find ways of connecting the personal to the political.*

Thinking About Democracy

The access course provided me with inspirational and challenging tutorials and a mandatory university application. My naivety was astounding in hindsight: I thought you could only study English, Math or Science at University! Then I remembered my dad shouting at the television saying that the study of Sociology was a 'mickey mouse' degree, so I opted for that on the basis that I might not be laughed out of the application stage. When I got the acceptance letter I was genuinely shocked—why would they let *me* go to university? When I later became University Admissions

Tutor I realised that getting a place at a 'new university' isn't that difficult, but for me, at that point in my life, it was like telling me I could go to Oxford. I accepted the place with excitement, pride and a whole new set of possibilities. I am eternally grateful to my access tutor who saw my enthusiasm for politics and advised me to switch course from Sociology to Politics, and to my Philosophy tutor (and now friend) for encouraging me to not only complete the BA degree but to go on and do an MA.

By the time I did my MA, I had three children and was making decisions about schools. The politics of choice was prevalent: Prime Minister Blair had been elected on the mantra of 'education, education, education'. I had worked in his telephone bank researching political intentions prior to the 1997 election and was interested in a form of direct democracy being introduced through referenda. He wanted the public to decide the future of grammar schools through a two-staged process of securing a referendum. It didn't prove very popular with the public despite it being part of Blair's commitment to a Third Way of governing a democracy. Bringing the best of right and left political thinking together in a new form of social democracy was supposed to appeal to the populace and refresh political dialogue. As I navigated the school admission process I wanted to understand more—my Masters dissertation title was decided: 'New Labour: Populism or Democracy?'

The study of politics and political decision making taught me about the machinery of government, but it was the study of political philosophy that not only made me think about the role of government and its relationship with the people it serves, but which literally changed my life again. I became committed to connecting the conversations that take place in communities with those that take place within the 'state'. Public Sector Plc (Local Government, Central Government, the Police and the NHS) was employing thousands of people and spending billions of pounds to serve people like me, but communities were becoming more passive and disengaged from politics.

Reviving civic life so that everyone might have a positive experience of being an active citizen seemed to me to be a necessity which ought to be invested in through both the formal routes (as was my experience of accredited courses), but also through the informal day to day interactions which enable the reawakening of the wonderful feminist phrase of 'the personal is political'. How could we show people that politics *does* affect their personal lives and that without healthy debate and positive engagement by 'ordinary' citizens we run the risk of democracy losing its way and being replaced by autocracy?

Acting Within a Democracy

Philosophers warn us of the risks to our imperfect system of government. Machiavelli argued that democratic government encourages corruption. For him, citizens who become indifferent to public affairs are, in effect, corrupt: he saw complacency and self-interested citizens as the greatest enemy of free government. Whilst I am not Machivellian, I find this difficult to argue with. However, unlike Machiavelli, I do believe democracy is worth fighting for which is generally my starting point in pursuing a better form of it to reflect our changing society.

In February 2014 the IPPR published 'Democracy in Britain: Essays in Honour of James Cornford' which captured the variety of ways in which the challenges facing democracy might be explored. Sarah Birch (2014) wrote about *inclusion* being the 'essence of democracy'. Recognising the imperfections in both the willingness of the public to engage in collective decision-making, and the translation by our institutions of the democratic ideal into the reality of politics, she still believes there has been a 'worrying *deterioration*' of the ability of our political system to include all citizens in the decision-making processes.

Studies show that alienation and trust are key contributing factors to the decline in participation. She refers to a study where it was found that the *words* politicians' use, as in not providing straight answers to questions, was more influential in determining their distrust of politicians than the misusing of official expenses and allowances (Birch 2014). This is important for public engagement and civic engagement generally, not just at election points. When thinking about reform Birch argues that our political and social institutions need to reframe:

- the way people see politics
- the incentives they have to engage with the political process; and
- their understanding of what they risk losing should they disengage

Birch cites the various reforms used to attempt to address this in recent years: Citizenship Education, flexible voting arrangements to encourage more convenient ways to vote, the Nolan principles of public life, Freedom of information, and debates about devolution. Yet as she points out, the average turnout for the UK Police and Crime Commissioners in 2012 was 15% and we still see low voter turnout at our local elections. She goes on to argue that there are four manageable ways to achieve the reframing of the above, outside some of the more challenging issues such as the links between political and social exclusion:[2]

- More robust citizenship education programmes;
- Lowering the voting age to 16;
- Make voting mandatory for first-time voters;
- A more determined approach to enforcing what is effectively compulsory electoral registration in the UK.

Recommendations 2–4 from above are of course all related to voting within the political system we have in the UK, and puts voting as the temperature gauge of the health of our democracy, but I think that is limited and misses the point of what she is trying to address. Democracy has to encourage the connection between the personal and political beyond the 2 min exercise of casting your vote. Citizens have to play their part in that if democracy is to flourish.

---

[2] See Birch in IPPR reference, but for a full analysis she signposts us to Allen and Birch.

Unlike Machiavelli, Tocqueville believed that '*the people who join with their neighbours to settle common problems and disputes will learn the importance of co- operation, feel a strong attachment to their community, and develop those habits of the hearts that led them to identify their own welfare with the welfare of the community as a whole*' (Ball et al. (2004).

But this doesn't just happen. We have a society that has lost faith in politicians, mistrusts the police and local government, and is increasingly questioning the honesty and integrity of those working in education and health. Voting once every 4 years has always felt like a democratic right that I would be willing to take to the streets for, but paradoxically it is also a minuscule part of what I believe our democratic reform should focus on. Building new relationships that connect the personal with the political are essential to refreshing democracy: we need new relationships between neighbours, and new relationships between the state and the individual. Relationships are central to developing trust; with good relationships we can achieve more together than we can alone.

Bourdieu, Coleman and Putnam are the founding fathers of thinking about relationships as 'capital'. Baron et al. (2010) summarise social capital simply as 'trust, norms and networks'. He argues that with these attributes in place, organisations can improve the efficiency of society by facilitating coordinated actions. He rightly (in my opinion) identifies a key barrier to this happening—people need to feel obliged to help each other, but how do we legislate for that obligation? We can't. We need to renew the social contract between the state and the individual by focusing on the social space that we inhabit collectively. Not through legislation and huge machinations of government, but by investing in communities to connect and engage in dialogue which brings the personal together with the political.

Social Capital achieves more than financial efficiencies—it creates places that feel safe, supportive and connected. The evidence is well documented in academia: Rosenfeld et al. (2001) produced findings that social capital had a significant effect on homicide rates, net of other predictors, while the unemployment and age composition of population had no effect. Coleman showed that social capital wasn't limited to the networks of the powerful, but 'conveyed real benefits to the poor and marginalised' (Baron et al. 2010, p. 23). Social capital arises out of trusting relationships between people who share assets such as knowledge and skills—knowledge and skills which the elected and unelected decision makers must learn to unleash and value.

The challenge for our democracy is how we build socially connected citizens who create their own social capital and value the democratic space they inhabit. By bringing the state and the individual together within a democratic social space we might bring politics closer to those who feel marginalised and disengaged. It is therefore the responsibility of the State within a democracy to nurture the right environment for those relationships to be built. The social, financial and political costs of not doing so will influence the future of our democracy, and our society in a negative way.

Institutional appetite for an asset-based approach to social policy is starting to develop, not just in the theoretical thinking but also in the willingness to invest in the practice. Some organisations' acknowledge that with the greatest will in the world, and significant funding, adopting a deficit model of public service delivery where we 'fix' communities rather than build on the strengths that they have, is just not working. Direct measurement of impact is however hard to measure and it often acts as a blockage to meaningful investment in communities. Norman (2010) warns us that *"releasing this energy is not a simple matter"* it is *"a monumental shift in culture"* (p. 196).

Changing the Culture of Democracy

Let's look at that culture. All governments must demonstrate their ability to serve the public well. Our recent history has shown the Blair and subsequent 'New Labour' governments measure this through the public confidence and satisfaction ratings of Public Services Plc. Citizens' Charters, pledges and Local Area Agreements were put in place to encourage organisations to check they were serving the community well. Partnership working became statutory for police and partners through Community Safety Partnerships. Engaged Communities was one of the hallmarks of success set out by the Home Office. Surveys were used to measure success through the levels of confidence and satisfaction of the public.

Targets distorted *practice*; rather than focusing on building relationships with the public, they built a huge machinery of officers and systems which looked for better ways of increasing *response rates* to surveys. I was part of a 'successful' Council programme which invested £60,000 in communications 'spin' just before the confidence and satisfaction surveys were conducted. We were praised for the manner in which we had successfully improved our relationship with the community, but we hadn't improved relationships, trust or norms, and we hadn't reduced demand on public services. We had managed to temporarily convince people that we were doing good work on their behalf, and as a result they should feel satisfied and confident in our services.

The problem with measuring success in that way is that branding and communication become key; police and other public services become preoccupied with their own messages and disingenuous in their approach to 'service' and social change. Laws and regulations become the norm, and enforcement the remedy for fixing 'bad' people. The New Labour governments during this period introduced an average of 3071 new laws per year under Prime Ministers Blair and Brown, set against a previous average of 1724 (Norman 2010).

When the coalition government took power in the UK they built on the learning from predecessors and the UK witnessed the birth of the new drive to build a Big Society. For Norman (2010), the Big Society is

> a set of interlocking ideas, even a philosophy: a concerted and wide ranging attempt to engage with the challenges of social and economic decline, and to move us towards a more connected society. It rests on the bold conjecture, that lying beneath the surface of British society is a vast amount of latent and untapped potential energy

Connecting that energy, so that we encourage a greater sense of cooperation, does indeed need a monumental shift in culture. It requires a much greater sense of co-operation between those serving the public and the public themselves. The gap between the state and the individual needs to change to reflect a greater commitment to cooperation and meaningful dialogue: the personal must become political, and the political must understand the eclectic nature of the personal.

Sennett (2012) argues that cooperation is a craft that we have lost over time. The 'good citizen' isn't so much about Aristotelian morality, but more a case of social competence in practical skills: good listening skills, being empathic, adopting a greater sense of curiosity, and following it up, are all positive characteristics of co-operation. Government with its laws and enforcement has arguably deskilled communities of those social competencies needed in a modern society to help manage aggression and improve the way we cooperate. With less cooperation and increased social incompetence (as in the skills above) it is no surprise that people revert to defensiveness and aggression at times. I have discovered over the last 15 years that those competences must be reflected in the practice of 'the state' itself if the state wishes to encourage them more widely in society.

It is indeed the 'fetish of assertion' which our parliament and public sector bodies display that demonstrates its discomfort with conversation and dialogue at a national and local level (Sennett 2012). We need to allow communities to define and measure what is important to them instead of imposing it to fit with the organisational need to compete with or blame other partners and/or to report to central government.

In her IPPR paper, Birch (2014) argued that to renew democracy we need a more robust approach to active citizenship in schools. Many years ago I agreed with her and was asked to co-lead a team of researchers who were looking for the evidence base for citizenship education. Sponsored by the Teacher Training Agency and the Evidence for Policy and Practice Information and Coordinating Centre (EPPI-Centre) we produced the first EPPI Systematic Review of the impact of citizenship education on the provision of schooling (Crick et al. 2004). This is what we found:

- **The quality of dialogue and discourse is central to learning** in citizenship education. Pedagogies need to be: facilitative; conversational; transformative; dialogical; and participatory.
- Teacher-pupil relationships need to be inclusive and respectful. Teachers may **need to 'let go of control'**. Students should be empowered to voice their views and gain meaning from their life experiences. Opportunities should be made for them to engage with values issues embedded in all curriculum subjects.
- **Contextual knowledge** can lead to citizenship engagement and action.
- A coherent whole-school strategy, including a community-owned values framework, is key. Participative and democratic processes in school leadership require particular attitudes and skills; schools **often restrict participation by students in shaping institutional practices while expecting them to adhere to policies.** Strategies for consensual change have to be identified by, and developed in, educational leaders.
- Teachers **need support to develop the appropriate professional skills**.

Replace the references to education and teaching with those to democracy and public servants and what you'll find is my challenge for our democracy. Ten years later, little has happened as a result of citizenship education because it wasn't valued in the curriculum: it was always the poor relation; the add-on subject rather than the foundation for all other curriculum subjects. Teachers received INSET days where they were given guidance on how to teach Citizenship but it varied: my children were taught that the Labour Party was the blue party and the Conservatives, red! These are very basic concepts which we expect our teachers to know, but are often untaught. Some of those teachers came from backgrounds like mine and would not have had the privilege of thinking about democracy and may not see the importance of it. We did see a lot of teaching of campaigning and protest (important for our democracy) but not much about cooperation, dialogue and social responsibility despite lesson plans and guidance encouraging them to do so.

It is a grim picture if we look at democracy through the deficit lens. But if we think about the richness in diverse 'private' lives across communities in the UK we might be able to breathe a huge kiss of life into our formal view of democracy.

The personal (for many) is not reflected in the political yet any observer of UK democracy could reasonably argue there is ample opportunity to participate in decision-making in between elections: it is on the face of it a good example of pluralism:

- 'Have your say' opportunities are in our local newspapers, bus stops, twitter, Facebook and so on;
- In a commitment to extend democracy in 2012, the coalition government gave the electorate in England and Wales an opportunity to democratize policing through the introduction of Police and Crime Commissioners;
- Every GP practice receives payment from the government to establish a Patient Participation Group to hear the public voice in health;
- Statute states that any significant changes to services must be consulted on in health in particular;
- The housing regulatory framework requires greater tenant engagement;
- Councillors are networking better with the rise of online social engagement;
- Residents can choose whether to have an elected mayor;
- Central Government has made petitioning easier on line;
- New laws around planning give communities the right to challenge and the right to build;
- A new Social Value Act aims to improve the social value added through contracting.

I could list so many opportunities 'offered' to the public by the State, but the fact remains that engagement outside moments of national crisis remains a challenge for the public sector. Without engagement we *waste* huge amounts of public money creating unsustainable 'solutions' to 'problems' which are defined by statistics and only show the surface of a situation.

Challenges to Meaningful Community Engagement

In the last 15 years I have taught potential teachers at degree and masters level, headed a service in local government committed to hearing the voice of local people, and managed programmes across the UK on behalf of the Home Office where we have explored how people choose to spend public money on listening to the voice of the public. Now I run MutualGain (www.mutualgain.org) which is designed to help support politicians, practitioners and the public to come together and build social capital.

Working with MutualGain has reinforced my view that without building the skills and experiences of active citizenship with all parties together we continue to offer 'projects' which won't be mainstreamed, and training which will be forgotten once the delegates have left the room. We at MutualGain deliver the reframing which Birch calls the way people see politics (politicians, practitioners and the public); the incentives they have to engage with the political process; and their understanding of what they risk losing should they disengage. Here are some anecdotes which typify the challenge we have ahead:

Politicians and Practitioners

Practitioners (*unelected* civil servants and local practitioners or policy makers) spend a significant length of time pacifying elected members. They often do what they can to keep elected members *away* from the business of governing the public. I can sometimes understand why they do this—the NHS reconfigurations of services are a good example in the UK at the moment where some elected representatives spearhead campaigns to 'save our hospital', mobilise tens of thousands of people to sign petitions to support the campaign despite clinicians concerns about the safety of patients in the hospital. One doctor recently described this to me as tantamount to 'killing a significant minority of his [the local MP's] constituents' but it goes down as a success if the building (not services) is saved.

When piloting the MutualGain model of building social capital with police, we came across politicians who wanted to stop us from talking to the public, and wanted us to work through just a select few residents who were known to them. They were vehemently opposed to incentivising the 'ordinary citizen' and felt they ought to value democracy as much as they did, and if they didn't, well they wouldn't get a say! This doesn't display the skills of letting go of control, and facilitation that the EPPI review required of teachers, and doesn't demonstrate the need for a new type of leadership which Christiansen and Bunt set out in their NESTA study in 2013.

Cast your mind back to when I was homeless with two children and poor, I didn't have time to engage in politics, but if the incentive was right and the experience was fun (see INVOLVE 2011), I could have brought assets of knowledge, skills and tactics to the table of policy makers and helped them serve me better.

The legitimacy of our public sector is under threat because of tokenistic consultation and engagement; confidence of the public is waning and trust is fast declining because of self-interested actors within the system itself (as much unelected as well as elected). Our public sector has become hard to reach for the public; it has lost its way when it comes to listening. It thinks that if it *tells* the public to engage, it will, but as so many public servants witness as they ask citizens to engage, they won't. The public needs to know that if they give up their time to share knowledge and resources, that there will be some return on investment. All too often the results of consultation and engagement sit in un-analysed boxes of surveys or are dismissed by those very servants who are not committed to democratic dialogue and participation.

Younge (2014) made the point in a guardian article about racism in the USA recently that '*the legal right of people to mix does not inevitably change the power relationship between them*'. The same can be said of democratic participation: The right to participate does not mean people will participate. Having the structures for engagement does not mean people will want to engage. Without participation the gap between the personal and the political will increase, discontent will grow and less desirable consequences could become more likely.

Conclusion

This personal journey has demonstrated to me the limitations of our 'democratic' institutions to adequately engage and understand those they serve; the unwillingness to share power between organisations to benefit those they serve, and the challenge of persuading the public to trust those who are there to serve them. If democratic government in the UK is founded on a social contract which permits 'representatives' to govern on our behalf, democracy is indeed in crisis. We can choose to focus on increased voter turnout, continue with under informed election campaigns, and use enforcement and law to fix the social problems we face. Or we could reframe the way we look at society and create public policy so that we connect the conversations taking place in communities with those in organisations so that we encourage a form of positive social capital to grow.

Community skills, knowledge and learning might prevent the gloomy predictions associated with what one local Council calls the 'graph of doom'[3], and a new form of social contract developed at a local level could reinstate the legitimacy of the state to govern us effectively. If the underlying principle of democracy is government for the people, of the people, by the people maybe we need to look beyond the formal mechanisms of 'representativeness' to discover what actually happens within society. Whether you are an advocate of direct democracy, participatory de-

---

[3] http://www.birmingham.ac.uk/Documents/college-social-sciences/government-society/inlogov/discussion-papers/new-model-discussion-paper−1012−2.pdf.

mocracy, deliberative democracy, consensus democracy, social democracy or indeed agonistic democracy the underlying principle and goal is the same.

I don't think I am arguing in favour of any specific brand of democracy, but rather calling for a refresh of the way in which we enact the social contract which underpins democracy in the UK. We need to build those skills outlined above when working within the state to develop social capital and we might lead by example and see a positive shift in our democracy.

References

Ball, T., Dagger, R., & O'Neill, D. (2004). *Political ideologies and the democratic ideal* (5th ed.). London: Pearson Education.

Baron, S., Schuller, T., & Field, J. (2010). *Social capital: Critical perspectives*. Oxford: Oxford University Press.

Birch, S. (2014). *Citizens excluded in democracy in Britain: Essays in honour of James Cornford*. London: Institute for Public Policy & Research.

Crick, R. D., Coates, M., Taylor, M., & Ritchie, S. (2004). *A systematic review of the impact of citizenship education on the provision of schooling*. London: EPPI-Centre, Social Science Research Unit, Institute of Education.

INVOLVE. (2011). *Pathways through participation: What creates and sustains active citizenship?* Final Report. London: Institute for Volunteering Research.

Norman, J. (2010). *The big society*. Buckingham: The University of Buckingham Press.

Rosenfeld, R., Baumer, E. P., & Messner, S. F. (2001). Social capital and homicide. *Social Forces, 80*(1), 283–310.

Sennett, R. (2012). *Together: The rituals, pleasures and politics of cooperation*. New York: Penguin.

Younge, G. (20 April 2014). On race, the US is not as improved as some would have us believe. *The Guardian*.

Susan Ritchie BA (Hons), MA (Research), MD designed the first undergraduate degree in Citizenship in the UK and co-authored the first EPPI Systematic Review of Active Citizenship (2004). After working for Tower Hamlets Council as Head of Governance and Participation for 6 years she was invited to lead on the Engaged Communities Hallmark of effective partnership working for the Home Office. She is now the Director of MutualGain which is an organisation established to support public sector workers connect more effectively with citizens. Having tested a range of new engagement techniques with a variety of so called 'hard to reach' groups, MutualGain is now testing a model of capacity building designed to support frontline staff, and the public, improve the way in which services are designed and delivered in the future.

Chapter 6
Dealing with Diversity in Police Services

Rowland Moore

Introduction

'Diversity in Policing'-a time hallowed theme about which much has been written and much discussed. It seems that not a week goes by before diversity related story hits the press. Some are positive, some not, but one thing is certain, they all seem newsworthy. So why, when the police service accepts the inherent need to represent the communities it polices, does it find it so difficult to manage diversity?

Kandola and Fullerton (1994) tell us that the basic concept of managing diversity accepts that the workforce consists of a diverse population of people. The diversity consists of visible and non-visible differences, which include factors such as sex, age, background, race, disability, personality and workstyle. "It is founded on the premise that harnessing these differences will create a productive environment in which everybody feels valued, where their talents are being fully utilised and in which organizational goals are met."

According to Rodgers and Hunter (1993), effective leadership in the twenty-first century requires that organisations acknowledge, implement and practice diversity management. Indeed, Syed and Kramar (2010) contend that organisations can achieve better business and equity outcomes associated with a diverse workforce by adopting a multilevel framework.

With under representation continuing to shackle modern day policing, how does a BME (Black Minority & Ethnic) police officer/Police Staff member fair? Being immersed in a culture dominated by people who aren't like you; be it by gender, sexuality, race or disability, presents significant additional personal challenges. However much one tries to 'fit in', they will always be noticed for their difference

R. Moore (✉)
Merseyside, Police, UK
e-mail: Rowland.Moore@merseyside.police.uk

© Springer International Publishing Switzerland 2015
P. Wankhade, D. Weir (eds.), *Police Services*, DOI 10.1007/978-3-319-16568-4_6

and that is where problems can develop. Some are obvious from the outset and are by definition easier to deal with whereas others are more insidious involving practices seemingly ingrained in organisational culture.

Policing Response to Diversity

Experience tells me that the overwhelming majority (of the majority) are genuine upright individuals. And yet from this position one can encounter major contradiction because the treatment of BME personnel does not consistently match the overt majority ideals. Prejudice, discrimination, unfairness, nepotism and racism thus pose a constant threat. Why?

The answer it seems, must lie in the culture of the organisation. This is where (like a tiny drop of yeast in a batch of dough), discrimination, prejudice and racism pervade, remaining (often dormant) in all areas of the organisation until activated by the 'enemy within'. Although numerically small in number, this group of pernicious individuals wield a hugely disproportionate influence to such an extent that their poison appears immovable. Why?

One of the most comprehensive studies on human values was that conducted by Milton Rokeach (1973). He argues that values reflect three characteristics- cognition, emotion and behaviour and that a person's value system is relatively stable and does not change substantially over time. He asserts that particular patterns of value orientation predict worldviews and thus can predict behaviour in the workplace. His survey instruments have been utilized in a USA policing context for over 40 years with surprisingly consistent results demonstrating validity.

A work place study of British police officers, utilizing the Rokeach Values Survey Instrument, demonstrated results consistent with those produced in similar studies in the United States. The study demonstrated a low ranking of the equality value item (16th out of 18 value items) and a high ranking of the freedom value item (joint 5th). The low ranking of the equality value and the high ranking of the freedom value correspond to Rokeach's (1973) two-value model of political orientation towards conservatism, which is consistent with previous studies conducted within police organisations.

The significance of this finding is that conservatism is a political philosophy or attitude emphasizing respect for traditional institutions, an inclination to maintain traditional order, distrust of government activism, and opposition to sudden change in the established order (Loftus 2010).

It is clear from the studies conducted in the United States (Rokeach et al. 1971; Sherrid 1979; Caldero and Larose 2001) that there is a value consistency among police officers spanning decades and geography. This has been echoed among British police officers (Loftus 2008, 2009 and 2010; Afful 2013). Thus the culture of police organisations may be perpetuated through this value structure.

Loftus (2010) asserts personal values significantly affect how an individual operates in the workplace and through ethnographic study, found a preference for political conservatism among British Police officers. "He also found an occupational culture that has remained fairly consistent over several decades shrouded in conservatism—a political philosophy or attitude emphasizing respect for traditional institutions, an inclination to maintain traditional order, distrust of government activism, and opposition to sudden change in the established order". This is magnified when Rodgers and Hunter (1993) state, "When the majority of the workforce shares similar backgrounds and experiences, and thinks, acts and looks alike, there is a level of certainty and predictability about workplace interactions." This goes some way to explain how the 'enemy within' perpetuate their influence.

Experience again shows that the genuine upright individuals who form the majority of policing create an inclusive atmosphere where meritocracy is the barometer and arbiter of success. The reality of modern racism is the institutional marginalisation of groups performed with the utmost discretion and minimum of fuss by a well versed, well educated, smart deadly minority. They remain the 'enemy within' strong and influential enough to dictate the pace of change the diversity agenda demands.

So where does this leave the BME Police Officer/Police staff member. How do they survive and achieve?

By accepting their difference, not trying to be someone else or something they are not and fully valuing themselves, they can inoculate against the enemy within. Achievement costs for any of us, none more so than when you are in the minority. Many talk of being 'tired'-Tired of working in an environment where you constantly feel tolerated as opposed to accepted; tired of working in an environment in which people have to be told how to behave; tired of having to prove yourself time and time again; and tired of fighting unconscious bias.

Psychologists tell us that our unconscious biases (being different about difference) are simply our natural people preferences. Biologically we are hard-wired to prefer people who look like us, sound like us and share our interests. Social psychologists call this phenomenon "social categorisation whereby we routinely and rapidly sort people into groups. This preference bypasses our normal, rational and logical thinking. We use these processes very effectively (we call it intuition) but the categories we use to sort people are not logical, modern or perhaps even legal. Put simply, our neurology can take us to the very brink of bias and poor decision making.

Neuro-psychologists tell us it is built into the very structure of the brain's neurons. Our unconscious brain processes and sifts vast amounts of information looking for patterns (200,000 times more information than the conscious mind). When the unconscious brain sees two things occurring together (e.g. many male senior managers) it begins to expect them to be seen together and begins to wire them together neurally. Brain imaging scans have demonstrated that when people are shown images of faces that differ to themselves, it activates an irrational prejudgment in the brain's alert system for danger; the amygdale. This happens in less than a tenth of a second. Our associations and biases are likely to be activated every time we encounter someone different to us, even if we consciously think that we reject a group stereotype. This massive discrepancy between our conscious and unconscious biases is the opportunity we have to improve our people decisions, and lever the advantages of talent for the benefit of our organisations.

Unconscious bias operates at a very subtle level, below our awareness. It results in almost unnoticeable behaviours (micro behaviours) such as paying a little less attention to what the other person says, addressing them less warmly or talking less to them. We tend to be less empathetic towards people who are not like us. These behaviours are small and not likely to lead to censure, but long-term exposure is corrosive.

Armed with this insight, Merseyside Police target their response in a number of ways. The Phoenix Leadership Programme led by Detective Inspector Afful, is a recruitment initiative aimed specifically at individuals with 'Protected Characteristics' as defined by the Equality Act 2010. Being under represented within the organisation, this group of individuals are invited to apply for the programme. They must be at least 18 years old and be prepared to join the Special Constabulary at the earliest opportunity. If successful at the application form/interview stage they are vetted. Subject to a positive result they are invited to attend an intensive week of inputs designed to increase knowledge of policing and raise personal confidence. This is followed by three workshops in the following 12 months relating to key areas of support i.e interview practice. Each individual is provided a mentor at the end of the week who will work with them for at least 12 months. To date, two separate cohorts of 15 and 10 individuals have successfully passed through the intensive week and 40 % of cohort 1 are now employed by the organisation.

A vibrant support network is another essential component in ensuring an equitable and inclusive working environment. Within Merseyside there are seven networks including Merseyside Black Police Association (MBPA). Existing to ensure fairness and equality for BME staff, MBPA enjoy a healthy and productive relationship with ACPO, PCC and senior management across the organisation. This engenders honest and open dialogue, something which is essential in assessing and unlocking the potential of BME staff. This is particularly important as fear still permeates the organisation with line managers wary to engage their BME colleagues as to how things are for them.

Mentoring and Sponsoring are key determinants in the retention and progression of BME officers with both types of support provided by the MBPA.

Conclusion

"In the final analysis, policing appears to be heavily populated by values underpinned in conservatism—a political philosophy or attitude emphasizing respect for traditional institutions, an inclination to maintain traditional order, distrust of government activism, and opposition to sudden change in the established order". Additionally, genuine upright individuals form the majority of policing creating an inclusive atmosphere where meritocracy is the barometer and arbiter of success. And yet the 'enemy within' remain a formidable foe seemingly able overhaul the majority with ease?

The answer seems to lie within unconscious bias fuelled by a conservative value system placing freedom/liberty above equality and favouring the status qou. If we can control and manage our unconscious biases it releases cognitive and emotional resources. These resources lead to better/fairer decision making and enhanced problem solving, increased ability to think in novel situations, better logical reasoning and more persistence.

Organisations need to help people create their own bias control trigger. If organisations create the right atmosphere where fairness is linked directly or indirectly to the organisation's goals, it can create the right conditions for a miss-match, which can trigger the individual's bias controls.

As a start, policing needs to consider where unconscious bias could have an impact i.e. in recruitment and promotion decisions, line management and performance appraisals. We need to consider training for all staff on what unconscious bias is and the impact it can have on their decision-making. Edmund Burke famously said '*The only thing necessary for the triumph of evil is for good men (people) to do nothing.*'

The challenge is to engender a change in values whereby the majority of genuine individuals hold freedom and equality in equal balance, thus accepting an upsetting of the status quo and subsequent paradigm shift!

References

Afful, I. (2013). A critical examination of how the values of equality and diversity are embedded within the organisational culture of Merseyside police to tackle ethnic minority under-representation: A case study of the force major incident team. Masters Dissertation, MSc in Police Leadership, Liverpool Hope University.

Caldero, M. A., & Larose, A. P. (2001). Value consistency within the police: The lack of a gap. *Policing: An International Journal of Police Strategies and Management, 24*(2), 162–180.

Kandola, R. S., & Fullerton, J. (1994). *Managing the mosaic—Diversity in action.* London: Chartered Institute of Personnel & Development.

Loftus, B. (2008). Dominant culture interrupted: Recognition, resentment and the politics of change in an English Police Force. *British Journal of Criminology, 48,* 756–777.

Loftus, B. (2009). *Police culture in a changing world.* Oxford: Oxford University Press.

Loftus, B. (2010). Police occupational culture: Classic themes altered times. *Policing and Society, 20*(1), 1–20.

Rodgers, J. O., & Hunter, M. (1993). Effective diversity management. *Handbook of Business Strategy, 4*(1), 222–227.

Rodgers, J. O., & Hunter, M. (2003). Effective diversity management. *Handbook of Business Strategy, 4*(1), 222–227.

Rokeach, M., Miller, M. G., & Snyder, J. A. (1971). The value gap between police and policed. *Journal of Social Issues, 27,* 155–171.

Rokeach, M. (1973). *The nature of human values.* New York: The Free Press.

Sherrid, S. (1979). Changing police values. In Speilberger, C. (Ed.), *Police selection and evaluation: Issues and Techniques* (pp. 167–176). New York: Hemisphere Publishing Corporation.

Syed, J., & Kramar, R. (2010). What is the Australian model for managing cultural diversity? *Personnel Review, 39*(1), 96–115.
Unconscious Bias fact sheet. (2014). Unconscious potential. www.ecu.ac.uk/events/materials/unconsious-bias-factsheet.doc. Accessed 28 Feb 2014.

Chief Supt. Rowland Moore (Rowley) has 28 years police service beginning his career with Essex Police in 1986. In December 1991 he was promoted to Sergeant and became a Chief Inspector in 2000. He got his promotion as Chief Superintendent in 2013 maintaining his role as head of Community Engagement in Merseyside Police. His input helped inform the debate on how to increase public confidence in Merseyside Police particularly by producing two reports-one related to the success in reducing the BRM Satisfaction Gap. The other put forward ideas on how to instill in staff, a commitment to act to increase community confidence in Merseyside Police. Rowley holds an M.A. and BSc in Social Science. A fully qualified Counsellor, he holds a Certificate and Diploma in Integrative Counselling as well as a Certificate in Cognitive Behaviour Therapy. In June 2014 he was awarded the YPAS 'Volunteer of the Year' Award. He is the Chair of the Merseyside Black Police Association. In 2013 he was nominated for the National Diversity Award (role model category) and also for the Black History Month Public Sector Award for services to community relations.

Chapter 7
Risk Management in Policing

Andrea Bishop

Context and Background

Risk management in policing is at the heart of everything that is carried out and it comes in different guises and is not always very clear. Strong leadership and operational credibility are crucial components for senior managers to readily possess and to successfully deliver against in policing. Confidence and trust of the public is an absolute priority and at the heart of British policing (Grieve et al. 2007). Members of the public will always turn to the police in times of need and it is in these difficult times that we must ensure that we get it right. This is what 'risk management' is all about. Maguire (2000, p. 315) argues about recent shifts in approaches to crime control, in particular the adoption of 'intelligence-led' policing strategies, and risk management techniques now evident at all levels, from transnational operations against organised crime, to local initiatives against persistent property offenders and even 'anti-social behaviour'.

From the moment I stepped out in uniform on patrol on the streets of Southampton 25 years ago, I started to learn about risk, from those around me and the situations I was presented with. What is it though? How does it present itself, how do you recognise it and how do you mitigate against it? This is just the beginning but what about then dealing with the personal responsibility of the cases you deal with, those that you investigate and those that you see through the court process and strive to deliver justice for the victims. What about the decisions you make as the senior officer in charge the consequences and the impact of those crucial decisions, the impact on a victim to the strategic risks?

A. Bishop (✉)
Kent, UK
e-mail: andrea.bishop@kent.pnn.police.uk

© Springer International Publishing Switzerland 2015
P. Wankhade, D. Weir (eds.), *Police Services*, DOI 10.1007/978-3-319-16568-4_7

Risk is so intangible yet it must be spelt out and fully explained, when teaching a new officer the skills they require. They of course must know about the powers and policies available to them but what they must learn so very quickly is how to recognise and deal effectively with new and emerging threats, harm and risk. They need to quickly understand the 'unseen risks' the 'what ifs' and learn to acquire the 'coppers nose' or 'gut feeling'.

But how do you go about teaching it? Some risks are clearly more obvious than others. For example, risk involved when the windows that are left open in a house providing easy access to a burglar, are easy to identify and provide the correct crime prevention advice. The domestic abuse situation where the victim has clearly been assaulted and the perpetrator is present, the risk can be evaluated. To leave a victim in an already hostile situation may mean that a reoccurrence of abuse is likely to happen; the risk may be assessed as 'high'. This is a risk that can be foreseen and therefore avoided if positive action is taken, such as an arrest or removal of the perpetrator (Maguire et al. 2001). The learning about risk management is quite clear which can be pointed out and taught in a way that is practical, operational and easy to apply with clear consequences anticipated. However, the risk is not always clear when the victim does not want to leave since the partner is the 'bread winner' and the request is primarily to stop the violence without the intention to leave. The risk management then becomes more complex and to simply do what the victim has requested leaves a greater risk to the victim once the police left the address/location.

Common sense plays a large part in risk management as in many situations it is about the ability to read a situation, take the right action to reduce or neutralise the risk entirely if possible. Equally, reducing the risk is better than taking no action at all, but the ability to identify the risk in the first place is the key. Therefore, we must 'reduce the risk, avoid the risk, remove the risk and finally accept it', which is a huge ask.

Risk is managed on a daily basis and decisions made within a police organisation will be scrutinised and hindsight is inevitably played out. In my view it provides the vehicle for managers to place themselves in the same situation to run through the information and see if they came up with the similar outcome. This is also done with the influence of others stating their opinions and in most cases seeing the result the decision has caused. This may appear obvious but it is fundamental in understanding risk management. Archbold (2005) has discussed how some of the largest law enforcement agencies in the USA use risk management in their efforts to control police liability.

I have worked in many different settings both as a detective and a senior commander and realised that experiential learning and exposure is fundamental to gaining that intuitive decision-making and tacit knowledge. This has provided me the ability to identify and evaluate the levels of risk. Yet this is hard to explain and articulate and the officer is not always sure how do you know when you have been successful as there might not always be a clear outcome.

For me, one of the most important skills but which is most under-estimated is that of listening. Listen carefully as to what is being said by those around you has helped me to understand the situation being presented more clearly. By proactive listening, we can assimilate the information provided (often under the media glare) and consider the threats and risks posed. This is relevant to policing in particular to understand the policy and powers available to deal with the risk and then consider (often very quickly) the tactical options that can be used to review the intelligence. Innes (2006) highlight the importance of community intelligence and democratic policing while responding to risks where the contours of the threat are uncertain. This is a model that is known and used every day and is referred to as the National Decision Model, (NDM). By following this model the right response is considered and rational decision making takes place (see Fig. 7.1).

There are six key elements of the NDM model. The pneumonic VIAPOAR acts as an aide-memoire in aspects of decision making:

- Values—Statement of mission and values
- Information—Gather information and intelligence
- Assessment—Assess threat and risk and develop a working strategy
- Powers and policy—Consider powers and policy
- Options—Identify options and contingencies
- Action and review—Take action and review what happened

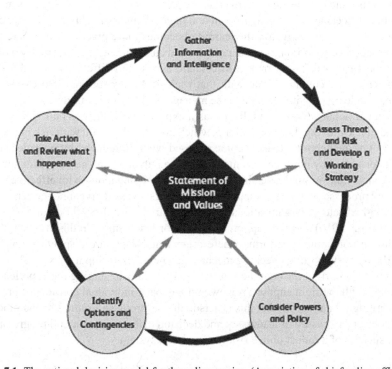

Fig. 7.1 The national decision model for the police service. (Association of chief police officers)

As already highlighted, the risks will present themselves in many different ways-both seen and unseen. An incident that has involved serious violence and immediacy may present very differently to an historical issue, but both may present the same risks and some actions may need a time-critical response. For example, a recent incident of serious sexual assault by an unknown perpetrator will require a great deal of care to be given to the victim, to capture best evidence and provide welfare support throughout the on-going investigation. Compare this to a historical sexual assault that comes to light years later, the same risk applies in the careful management of that victim. The evidence is clearly still sought with the same rigour and professionalism. Good risk management is also about the approach of the officer involved and the actions taken. Each person has a reasonable expectation of what should happen next and what the police should do. Investigation appropriate to the crime involved should include following up the reasonable lines of enquiries and sharing the progress of the investigation with the victims as allowed under the law. The authenticity and integrity of the decision making is paramount and adds to the credibility of the decision making, particularly if scrutinised. Ratcliffe's (2008) notion of 'intelligence-led' policing is similarly predicated on the premises of a sound risk management system.

The risk is presented in many ways with all; some or none may surface at some point in the investigation. Dealing with organisational and force reputational risk, personal risk and a very public media risk are part of daily policing. Decisions made by police officers are clearly significant and hugely important. Having experienced many cases as an investigator, the learning becomes more practiced. It is here the rank structure comes into its own in policing and compliments the system. By working at the various different ranks, officers are exposed to different risk and threat levels which are commensurate with that rank. It is only through that exposure, sharing and learning with others that the management of risk is improved over time. Operational policing is fast and diverse as it exposes individuals to both time-critical and quick-moving decision making, which goes hand in hand with risk management as outlined above. Risks become exposed when introduced by poor decision makers or stifled by non-decision makers. Those outcomes can be very damaging.

In conclusion, strong leadership is required in policing along with effective systems and processes in place to support operational business. This cannot be achieved by individuals alone. Organisations can only flourish with the right culture (Foster 2005; Loftus 2010) and the support of the senior leadership. Credibility, visibility and strong operational platforms where brevity and depth are displayed, coupled with the right supportive checking mechanisms help to develop a strong risk management system right through the organisation which help sharing the experiential learning. With the right support, review and feedback individual confidence grows and learning is banked whether this is personally or through a forum. The incremental phases and exposure of leadership and decision making are a natural progression to the success of a robust police risk management system.

References

Archbold, C. A. (2005). Managing the bottom line: Risk management in policing. *Policing: An International Journal of Police Strategies & Management, 28*(1), 30–48.

Association of Chief Police Officers. (2014). The national decision model. http://www.acpo.police.uk/documents/president/201201PBANDM.pdf. Accessed 18 Sept. 2014.

Foster, J. (2005). Police cultures. In T. Newburn (ed.), *Handbook of policing*. Cullompton: Willan

Grieve, J., Harfield, C., & MacVean, A. (2007). *Policing*. (SAGE Course Companions series). London: Sage.

Innes, M. (2006). Policing uncertainty: Countering terror through community intelligence and democratic policing. *The ANNALS of the American Academy of Political and Social Science, 605*(1), 222–241.

Loftus, B. (2010). Police occupational culture: Classic themes altered times. *Policing and Society, 20*(1), 1–20.

Maguire, M. (2000). Policing by risks and targets: Some dimensions and implications of intelligence-led crime control. *Policing and Society: An International Journal of Research and Policy, 9*(4), 315–336.

Maguire, M., Kemshall, H., Noaks, L., & Wincup, E. (2001). Risk assessment and management of known sexual and violent offenders: A review of current issues. National Criminal Justice Reference Service. https://www.ncjrs.gov/App/Publications/abstract.aspx?ID=201585. Accessed 30 Sept. 2014.

Ratcliffe, J. H. (2008). *Intelligence-led policing*. Cullompton: Willan.

Supt. Andrea Bishop joined Hampshire Constabulary in 1989 and was stationed in Shirley in Southampton. In 1992 she transferred to Kent Police where she spent many years on local divisions gaining experience in CID and Public Protection becoming a career detective. Moving up through the ranks she continued in Divisional and Specialist Crime. More recently, as Superintendent she has gained experience in the tactical arena, training as a Firearms and Public Order Commander and now works as Deputy Divisional Commander in the East of the County.Author Query

Chapter 8
Perspectives on the Essence of Policing

Jon Murphy

Context and Background

I will aim to deliver a meaningful state of the nation on British Policing and Merseyside Police in particular. I think it is best to deliver a wide-ranging look across the piste, rather than examine a particular aspect of policing. It is, I think, a particularly interesting juncture to do this.

Before I talk about policing, I thought I would say a few words about the great city of Liverpool and its people. The transformation has been nothing short of miraculous and despite austerity the city is holding its own. It is a hugely different city from the one I encountered when I first walked the beat. I remember, as if it was yesterday, walking out of Copperas Hill Police Station to the smell of the breweries, the run down city centre, a derelict Albert Dock and dilapidated 1930's tenement blocks. But now, the symbols of regeneration are all around us—Liverpool One, new museums and galleries, hotels, restaurants, the Echo arena. But whilst the landscape of the city has changed the heartbeat has not, the spirit of the people is indomitable. The sense of humour, talent, resilience and sense of community have all been central to transformation. Despite these difficult times I have no doubt that the city will continue on its resurgent path. Merseyside Police has a central part to play in this in keeping communities' safe, continuing to reduce crime and working with the councils, the academic institutions and all other partners to make Liverpool and the county of Merseyside a safe place to live, to work, to study and an attractive place to invest.

An early version of this chapter was presented at the Liverpool John Moores University in October 2013

J. Murphy (✉)
CC Merseyside Police, Merseyside, UK
e-mail: chief@merseyside.pnn.police.uk

© Springer International Publishing Switzerland 2015
P. Wankhade, D. Weir (eds.), *Police Services,* DOI 10.1007/978-3-319-16568-4_8

In 1829 Sir Robert Peel laid out his 9 principles of the modern police including the often quoted statement that 'the police are the public and the public are the police'. I believe that in Merseyside this maxim is epitomised. We are as much a part of Merseyside's communities as the people we are charged with keeping safe—in short we care! I am immensely proud to be the Chief Constable of the force I joined as a 16 year old cadet on 6th January 1975—almost 39 years ago. I am immensely proud to be Chief Constable of the city I was born and raised in and indeed the first local born chief Merseyside Police has ever had. My father before me was a Liverpool City Police officer so I guess I have known little else. In 1982 I entered the CID now 'Life on Mars' is billed as a comedy drama had it been made when I was a young detective it would have been a 'fly on the wall' documentary! Other than an all too brief 12 months as a uniform sergeant I spent the next 18 years as a detective, rising to become a Senior Investigating Officer responsible for homicide, corruption and every other type of serious crime investigation that Merseyside can throw at a detective. I have no intention of cataloguing my whole career. I simply characterise my own policing background here in Liverpool to demonstrate how it has shaped my understanding of the communities of Merseyside and the challenges my officers face.

The job itself is demanding but never dull, no 2 days are the same and every day officers and staff do fantastic things. My correspondence is a never-ending tide of deep joy and from time to time the odd gem does come across my desk. I recently received a letter from a member of the public thanking me for the compassion and understanding extended to her by a family liaison officer during a critical incident. She wrote and I quote 'he has more balls than any man I have ever met. He took on my mother-in-law and won!! This is a feat that has never even been tried, let alone won, in all the years I have known her'.

Policing in the Era of Austerity

The Police service has always been excellent at training its people; we invest huge amounts of money and resource in training our people in how to do stuff, about the law, codes of practice, about process and about tactical delivery. But whilst we train well, what we are not so good at is teaching our people to think about policing, about the mission and about legitimacy.

Her Majesties Chief Inspector of Constabulary, Tom Winsor, in his report (2012) into police terms and conditions lamented the police service not being a profession. I should point out he is the first non-police officer in 150 years to perform the role. Nonetheless whilst he may lament, I would suggest that most of the police officers in this country do regard themselves as professionals, me included. But this is clearly not how he sees us and neither, it would appear, do government. So, if we truly want to be professionals and regarded as such then, in my view, we need to foster a much greater understanding in our junior and middle ranking officers in the more philosophical questions about policing at a much earlier point in service and not wait until officers attend senior command training when for better or worse the die is cast.

This more philosophical study allied to quality training in professional skills is, I think, the key to a professional police service. So what are these philosophical questions that warrant such attention? Here are some starters:

- What do we mean by legitimacy and policing by consent?
- Does legitimacy come from what we do or how we do it?
- What exactly is the policing mission?
- Is what we think the mission is the same as what the public think?
- How far should the state (in the form of the police) be able to intrude into people's private lives in order to protect the wider public?

In a recent speech on policing to the 'Reform' think-tank, the Police Minister Damian Green (Hope 2013) opened thus:

> The job of cleaning out the stables is key

Now we all know what is found in the stables and this is perhaps an unfortunate metaphor for the necessary exercise of getting into the public domain what should have been there in the first place. But nonetheless, the use of the metaphor does serve to reflect the damage to the service's reputation and the precarious and uncertain position we find ourselves in—as a consequence of largely, but not exclusively, historic failures.

The terrible tragedy of Hillsborough is, without doubt, a watershed and I say 'is' rather than 'was' because we are only at the start of a journey that will last for some considerable time yet as the families rightly seek justice and the truth unfolds (Hillsborough Report 2012; Hughson and Spaaij 2011). Hillsborough has had a domino effect in informing government and contemporary public opinion of the police as successive bad news stories have unfolded in the media. The Leveson Enquiry, 'Plebgate', the first Chief Constable in over 30 years to be sacked, failings in child sexual abuse investigations, undercover officers fathering children, and other stories in the media (Public Administration Select Committee 2014) are understandably being viewed through the lens that is Hillsborough: that the police tell lies and the police are corrupt.

I make no comment about the rights and wrongs of any of these stories. I simply illustrate that individually and collectively they have been immensely damaging. I genuinely can't remember when the police service felt so under siege and I certainly can't recall such a feeling of impotence and inability to influence change for the better. This is happening at a time when the service is going through the biggest reform since Sir Robert Peel. All of this has coincided with the election of Police and Crime Commissioners, many would argue with little or no prior knowledge of policing beyond what they, like everybody else, read in the papers. Their election came within weeks of the Hillsborough report (2012) and closely coincided with the Lord Leveson enquiry (www.levesoninquiry.org.uk), an Inspectors of Constabulary report into police integrity (HMIC 2011) and the Saville revelations (ITV 2012), a powerful cocktail to influence Police and Crime Commissioners' (PCCs) opinions of the service for which they are now accountable to the public. It would be odd if this were not to give them a particular view of the world, particularly as regards the leadership of the service. Put simply, the question posed, can I trust my Chief Constable?

But as challenging as all of this is, it is a fact of life in our democracy so in my view, best we get on with it. I need to help my young officers make sense of it all and focus on the job in hand. So what about policing on Merseyside?—What are our priorities, how well are we doing and how is life with the Commissioner? Put simply, our job is to fight crime and protect our communities or in the parlance of our force vision to deliver 'Excellent Policing' for the communities of Merseyside. But of course it isn't simple. The policing mission is broad, complex and demanding, 24/7,365 days a year.

Relationships with PCCs

I am also conscious that many of my Chief Constable colleagues are experiencing a very different kind of relationship. It is still very early days and certainly too early to make any judgement on whether the system, as opposed to individual Chief/PCC relationships, is an improvement on what we had before. One or two examples of a relationship working well, can no more be an endorsement of the system than one or two working not so well can draw a very different conclusion. Only time will tell.

The police are very much the agency of last resort with more than a third of all incidents we respond to on a daily basis being social work rather than crime related. As a young officer I was very much in the police *force* as opposed to the police *service* camp. As you get older and (I hope) wiser you realise that enforcement is no solution to anything; it delivers short to medium term respite at best. As Peel identified almost 200 years ago, the test of the police will be the absence of crime: Prevention is better than cure. Despite public perception, crime on Merseyside is down 13 % in the last 3 years. Merseyside is a safe place to live and work. But we see dramatic headlines relating to gun crime and this continues to be a challenge and a cause for great concern. But whilst high impact, these events thankfully remain very few in number and are on a downwards trend. It is not the crime statistics that matter; it is our relationship with the public and the fact that the public consistently have more confidence in Merseyside Police than nearly every other police force in the country. Despite the depressing national picture, our local relationship is intact.

Philosophy of Police Leadership

I now turn to my passion and what I have referred to as my philosophy of policing. Despite my philosophy descriptor there is nothing revolutionary or clever about it, quite the opposite! I don't believe in fixing what is isn't broken and I don't believe in change for change sake. That said, austerity has forced Merseyside Police to negotiate the most comprehensive and complex change programme it has ever gone through. Despite that, the basic leadership philosophy holds good; 'Keep it simple' (at least as simple as I can), talk to the staff (and for that matter the public) in straightforward simple language, be honest with people, give the staff a bit of tough love (with emphasis on the love) and appeal to their emotions. People want to work towards something they believe in, not simply to do what they are told. To have pride in the badge they wear, the organisation they belong to, the job they do and the communities they police. Whilst what we do is important, it is '*how we do it*' that really matters and predominately influences public opinion.

In August 2011 Liverpool experienced significant disorder. The officers of Merseyside Police did a fantastic job in protecting the public and property. But the striking element of that success was the overwhelming public support they received in Toxteth in particular. Community leaders mobilised, mediated with young people intent on rioting, fed and watered tired and exhausted officers and came out to support the Mayor in cleaning up. That was a fantastic endorsement for Liverpool's community spirit. There is nothing new in the concept of engendering public support through doing things the right way: policing by consent.

I have a copy of a speech delivered by the Head Constable of Liverpool to a group of new recruits in 1862, other than urging his men to find a good wife who could darn socks! His words stand good today. He talks of a Constable of rough disposition and one of an altogether smoother disposition and their different approaches to dealing with a young boy flying a kite in a busy roadway as horses pass by. The constable of rough disposition snaps the boy's kite over his knee and puts him before the magistrate. This will never do, the Head Constable exclaims! He then talks of the constable of smooth disposition who gently points out to the boy the danger of scaring horses and that he should take his kite to the field and so demonstrating, he states that 'the constable has regard for what the public may think of him'. He concluded that 'the opinion of the public is often formed by the single act of a single individual'. The Head Constable was a man of great vision who recognised that the key to success is, in the language of today, the culture of the organisation—how we do our job in a way that engenders public support and thereby enables us to police by consent.

The culture in any organisation is determined by its leadership. I am very conscious that it is me that sets the tone and rhythm of the force and ultimately the culture—and it is a responsibility I take very seriously. I take every opportunity I can to talk to the officers and staff of the force—with all the demands of the job it is not as easy as it sounds. When I do talk to them I make absolutely clear what I expect of them:

- Courtesy and respect—there is no excuse for incivility.
- Professional competence—the ability to keep the public safe and to solve their problems
- Absolute integrity—you only lose it once!

- To use their powers for the right reason—not because they can or to satisfy some meaningless statistical return.
- Humility—We all make mistakes—apologise, put things right and move on!
- Humility extends to me!
- Compassion—the human touch and a sense of humour!—it's ok to have a laugh at work and enjoy yourself!
- To land the message—'how we do things' I have adopted three simple but powerful themes—Just Talk—Just Think and Just Lead.
- Just Talk—talking to the public whenever we can and wherever we can—not just because a person is a victim, a witness, being arrested or given a ticket—Provided it is appropriate I don't care what they talk about—'is the kettle on',"how are the kids" or even a joke—Just talk to people. If we don't talk to the public, they won't talk to us.
- Just Think—my officers do their job in a goldfish bowl, on CCTV and in the full glare of the media -never have standards of behaviour and values been more important in delivering both a professional service and the forming of positive opinions.

Despite the failings of a few, I have no doubt that standards are higher than they have ever been. I have made it clear that bad behaviour will not be tolerated. It is painful to wash your dirty linen in public but if that is what it takes to get people out of the organisation when they don't live up to our standards then that is what we will do.

From the minute the most junior officer walks out of a police station they are looked upon by the public as a leader. The public do not differentiate rank or experience. All they see is a uniform and they look to it for help and to have their problems solved. Leadership and holding rank is not the same thing though I should say we do endeavour to have the two things coincide. For the most part rank happens in the police station, the decisions, judgements and actions of our most junior officers require leadership skills of the highest order. Sometimes they involve life and death and they are always a crisis for somebody.

If you ask any of my senior officers what is the most important factor in selection for promotion in Merseyside Police, I guarantee they will all give the same answer: being a leader and professional competence—the 2am test, when a crisis happens can this individual keep the public safe and protect our reputation. We maintain and build on our reputation by keeping the public safe, not by obfuscation or being risk averse but by running towards danger when others are running away and by being openly accountable for our actions.

Policing in Austerity

Also the reality of the ongoing reduction in the forces budget cannot be entirely ignored. Since I became Chief in January 2010, the force has lost around 1000 people. 700 less police officers, the rest police staff. I suspect more will have to leave over the next 3 years and probably beyond. We have to get on with it and do our best for the public. But the challenge of ongoing austerity is not just about balancing the books; it is about re-engineering the organisation and transforming the way we deliver our services. There continues to be a political and public obsession with visibility—re-assurance enshrined in the neighbourhood policing model irrespective of actual neighbourhood demand propped up by the pursuit of numerical targets to measure neighbourhood against neighbourhood and force against force.

But how long can we sustain this model and style of policing? Which is more important-deploying resources in big hats and high visibility jackets to make the public feel safe or focusing on what is less visible to the public but actually does protect them from the more serious threats of child sexual abuse, cyber crime, serious organised crime, hate crime and many, other disciplines requiring a specialist response. Should we focus all of our efforts on the identification of threat, harm and risk and allocate resources accordingly? This is controversial stuff I know. Whilst we all like to see a bobby, the vast majority of the public don't need a visible police presence and they will only ever call for service once or twice, if ever, over many, many years. Perhaps we should be more realistic about what we can offer them when they are not calling us for help.

Those of a certain generation can remember when if you were sick the doctor might come to the house. That rarely happens any more. I don't see fire fighters, paramedics or nurses walking the streets in case somebody becomes ill or to reassure those of us who are actually quite well but like to see them around. Flippant I know and I am not making the case for any particular resource allocation model, but there is a serious point—what commercial organisation would take approaching 25 % out of its budget and keep trying to deliver the same services? This does not mean that I don't believe in Neighbourhood Policing. In fact to date the numbers of Merseyside officers working in neighbourhood teams has remained the same despite the cuts.

But what I do believe and instil in staff is that the whole force is actively engaged in Neighbourhood Policing in whatever function or specialist role an individual happens to be, not just those officers on dedicated neighbourhood teams. Visibility alone is too simplistic. True neighbourhood policing is about the relationship all members of the force have with the public whether a neighbourhood officer, a detective, a PCSO or whatever. Neighbourhood Policing is not about structure or even resource allocation, it is about how we listen to the public, how we speak to people, how we solve their problems when they need us and delivering on our promises. Put simply, it is *not what we do but how we do it*.

Conclusion

So to conclude, what does the future of policing hold? It is not just austerity that presents a threat to the delivery of local policing. What of socio-economic and technological changes over which the police have no influence such as:

- The globalisation of markets for goods and services
- The advent of fast communications, new social media and the increasing pace of technological change.
- New crimes committed in new ways
- Economic and social migration—new communities with different needs and bringing new challenges.
- Growing income inequality
- The fragmentation of families and old established communities

All of these things will bring the police service new challenges. I have no doubt we will rise to them like we have always done. In the meantime we will continue to continually re-engineer the organisation making sure we are fit for purpose and we identify and manage risk. We should focus on the job in hand that 'we are here to serve' and we will continue to deliver an excellent policing service. And we should try to build for a better future. Despite austerity I have the privilege of leading a body of fantastic people. I tell them that every chance I get. I tell them that we have an outstanding reputation hard won over almost 200 years. I rather like the slogan of a rather expensive watch company:

'You never actually own one of their watches—you look after it for the next generation'

That is what I tell my officers on the day they join and remind them at every opportunity that the safety of the public and the reputation of Merseyside Police is in their hands and they should guard them both well. I am quite proud to say that THEY GET IT!

References

Her Majesty's Constabulary of Inspection. (2011). *Without fear or favour: A review of police relationships*. London: HMIC.

Hughson, J., & Spaaij, R. (2011). You are always on our mind: The Hillsborough tragedy as cultural trauma. *Acta Sociologica, 54*(3), 283–295.

Hillsborough Independent Panel. (2012). *Hillsborough The Report of the Hillsborough Independent Panel*. HC 581. The Stationery Office Limited: London.

Hope, C. (2013). Police should be more polite to the public, says policing minister Damian Green. *The Telegraph*. Published 8 July 2013.

ITV. (2012). *Exposure: The other side of Jimmy Savile*.

Public Administration Select Committee. (2014). *Caught red-handed: Why we can't count on Police Recorded Crime statistics*. Thirteenth Report of Session 2013–14. HC 760. The Stationery Office Limited: London.

Sir Jon Murphy QPM, Chief Constable joined Merseyside Police as a Cadet in January 1975. After early uniform roles in Toxteth and Liverpool city he spent 3 years in the force support group, during which time he was on the front line of the 1981 Toxteth riots. Shortly after the riots he entered the CID as an aide and there followed an almost 20 year unbroken career as a detective, rising to the rank of Detective Superintendent SIO. He left Merseyside to join the National Crime Squad as Assistant Chief Constable, Head of Operations in 2001. He returned to Merseyside Police in 2004 as Deputy Chief Constable. In February 2010 he took up his current position as Chief Constable of Merseyside Police. He has read Law at Liverpool University and has a postgraduate Criminology Diploma from Cambridge. Sir Jon has been commended on 14 occasions and was awarded the Queen's Police Medal in the 2007 Birthday Honours. In 2012 he was given a Lifetime Achievement Award by the Police Federation National Detective Forum and in 2013 he was voted Mersey Region Public Sector Leader of the Year. In 2014 he received a Knighthood in the Queen's Birthday Honours.

Part III
Current Debates in Policing

Chapter 9
Enhancing Police Accountability in England and Wales: What Differences are Police and Crime Commissioners Making?

John W. Raine

Introduction

The election across England and Wales on November 15th 2012 of 41 Police and Crime Commissioners (PCCs)—one for each police force area outside London (where the equivalent functions had already been vested in the Mayor of London)—marked the launch of an intriguingly novel approach to police governance at the local level. Replacing the tradition of committee-style governance, originally of council-led 'police committees', and subsequently (from 1964) of separate 'police authorities' (comprising a mix of nominated councillors and other local appointees), the new PCCs are directly-elected individual office-holders whose role it is to provide the strategic leadership and democratic governance for police and crime-related activity, including the key role of holding the chief constable and the local police force to account on behalf of the public (Raine and Keasey 2012).

The idea for PCCs arose amidst general disappointment with the apparent dearth of impact of police authorities and in particular, with their very low public profile. The New Labour government considered various options for strengthening police governance as part of its wider plans for policing reform (Home Office 2008) but failed to identify a satisfactory way forward. So it fell to the incoming Conservative/Liberal-Democrat Coalition government in 2010 to take up the challenge. The idea of directly-elected police and crime commissioners had been proposed some 8 years earlier by the Conservative Member of Parliament, Douglas Carswell. A

This chapter is a specially edited version of a longer chapter 'Electrocracy with Accountabilities? The Novel Governance Model of Police and Crime Commissioners', in Lister S and M Rowe (eds) (2015) *Policing and Accountability,* London: Routledge.

J. W. Raine (✉)
Institute of Local Government Studies, University of Birmingham, Birmingham, UK
e-mail: j.w.raine@bham.ac.uk

© Springer International Publishing Switzerland 2015

P. Wankhade, D. Weir (eds.), *Police Services,* DOI 10.1007/978-3-319-16568-4_9

strong advocate of localism and of direct democracy, Carswell was keen to replicate in this country the kind of police governance arrangements he understood to operate well in US cities. In fact, however, the model of police and crime commissioners that he proposed to his political party was rather different from that of US city police commissioners—who are either professional police officers (equivalent to chief constables in the UK) or experienced administrators, rather than elected politicians.

But three other factors were influential in ensuring that the new Coalition Government's initial policy prospectus included a commitment to: '*introduce measures to make the police more accountable through oversight by a directly elected individual, who will be subject to strict checks and balances by locally elected representatives*' (H M Government 2010, p. 13). First, was the growing enthusiasm in both national and local political circles for the idea of 'commissioning' public services, and for greater plurality in the pattern of provision as a result of contracting with private and third sector organisations as an alternative to the traditional dominance of 'in-house' public provision (Bovaird et al. 2013). Second, was strong interest of the Coalition Government in the polity of 'new localism' and the desire to end the extent of centralisation that had come to be seen as a defining hallmark of the preceding New Labour government, although, as Lowndes and Pratchett (2012) noted, the roots of 'new localism' were already well established in Labour's developing 'communities agenda'. Third, was the Government's enthusiasm (as indeed that of New Labour) for directly-elected leaders at local level, particularly for the more decisive and efficient form of decision-making that they were presumed to invoke. While the efforts to persuade councils and local public opinion in favour of the concept of directly elected mayors had proved largely in vain, with very few local authorities taking up the option, the reform of police governance was seen by the Coalition Government as an opportunity to introduce across the country the essential elements of the model—of directly-elected individual office-holders—albeit specifically for policing.

Unfortunately, the Government's enthusiasm for the new model was hardly matched in wider circles. The relevant clauses of the Police Reform and Social Responsibility Bill 2012, introducing PCCs were opposed by a number of Conservative and Liberal-Democrats as well as by the formal opposition parties in both the House of Commons and Lords; there was outspoken criticism of the proposals by several chief constables and much scepticism among the wider policing and criminal justice practitioner community, and the turn-out of voters at the first elections on 15th November 2012 averaged just 14.7%—a record low for a nation-wide ballot, reflecting a mix of ignorance, confusion and disinterest in the idea of PCCs on the part of the eligible voting public. For a while afterwards, moreover, matters seemed to get worse for the Government as a succession of negative media headlines added to the embarrassment about the elections. Such headlines included allegations of cronyism, as several PCCs sought to appoint their election assistants to leading roles within their offices; unexpected costs to the public purse associated with recruitment of teams of staff; and tensions and disagreements with chief constables, in more than one case, involving attempts at dismissal (Laville 2013).

It all amounted to a particularly inauspicious start for England and Wales' new police governance model, and while after just 1 year, it seemed unreasonably premature of the Independent Police Commission to describe the PCC model as '*systemically flawed as a method of democratic governance*' and to recommend its abolition (IPC 2013, p. 81), such a conclusion was symptomatic of the on-going doubts about the Coalition's bold initiative.

This chapter does not set out to conclude one way or the other about the case for PCCs, nor indeed to offer any definitive assessment of the model and of its overall effectiveness. Instead it focuses on one particular aspect; one which was especially prominent in the minds of the early advocates—that of the impact of accountability in policing. In so doing, the chapter seeks to take stock of what the introduction of PCCs has thus far meant in this respect, and in relation to various potentially significant accountability relationships. In fact five such relationships are examined: accountability of PCCs to the public; accountability in relation to the Police and Crime Panels (established in each police area as a scrutiny body to hold the Commissioner to account on behalf of the public); accountability to central government and the Home Secretary in particular (given that the relevant legislation also refers to each PCC's responsibility to provide for the national 'strategic policing requirement'); accountability of PCCs towards their sponsoring political parties (where such sponsorship is provided); and, conversely, accountability of chief constables towards their PCCs[1].

These five accountability relationships are highlighted in Fig. 9.1 with the shaded arrows, though, as can be seen, the diagram also indicates other relationships of potential significance albeit without the element of direct accountability, notably in relation to community safety partnerships, local criminal justice boards and providers of criminal justice services.

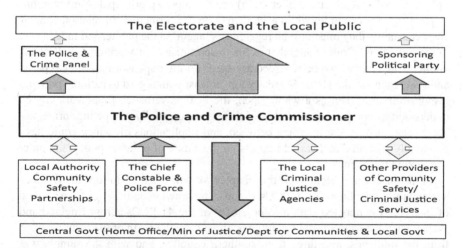

Fig. 9.1 PCC relationships and accountabilities

---

[1] Space here does not permit inclusion here, but several additional accountability relationships for PCCs are further explored in Raine (2014).

Principal-Agent Theory and Research on PCC Accountability Relationships

In examining such accountability relationships, it is helpful to draw on Principal-Agent Theory from the discipline of economics, and which has been much discussed and applied in seeking to understand motivation and behaviour in inter-relational settings (see for example: Mayston 1993; Wood and Waterman 1994; Waterman and Meier 1998; Besley 2006; Bertelli 2012). This is theory that focuses, in its most simple form, on the relationship between the 'commissioner' of a task (or service provision activity)—'the principal'- and the 'contractor' who undertakes the work—'the agent'. A familiar problem in such situations, however, is that the agent (as contractor) will often know rather more about the tasks involved than the 'principal'—the problem of 'information asymmetry' as it is usually described (Ferris and Graddy 1998; Bandyopadhyay 2013)—and may well seek to exploit that superior knowledge to their own advantage, for instance, by suggesting a larger-scale job than is really needed, and/or by charging more than is reasonable. The key challenge, then, for the 'principal' is to ensure that appropriate checking processes and incentive arrangements are in place to ensure that the interests of the commissioner are protected and the contractor does not exploit the situation. Carrying this general line of thinking into police governance, then, for example, a key question might concern the means by which a directly-elected PCC can be confident that their chief constable and police force (as agent) is indeed addressing each of the locally-decided policing priorities to the best of their abilities, and not just focusing on those to which, as professional officers, they happen also to be committed.

Moreover, the situation with police governance, (as indeed, in many public service contexts) can often prove more complex still because of the problem of 'multiple principals' (Knott and Miller 2006) or of competing principal-agent relationships. Thus, for example, while a PCC may be the 'principal' in relation to their chief constable, they must also be regarded as 'agent' to the public, and indeed also to the Police and Crime Panel that exists to scrutinise their work on behalf of the public. A PCC may also be regarded as 'agent' to their sponsoring political party, and also 'agent' to the Home Secretary too, at least with regard to national policing responsibilities. Taken as a whole, then, the PCC governance framework can be understood as comprising a number of different, potentially competing, principal-agent relationships, the interplay between, and implications of, which could have potentially profound and varied impacts on the nature of policing policy and practice around the country.

In the succeeding sections of this chapter we will consider in turn the five key accountability relationships of PCCs, doing so by drawing on findings from a round of interviews conducted with a sample of 9 of the 41 PCCs across England and Wales. The nine were selected as follows: three from the north of the country; three from the midlands, and three from southern counties, and with the sample was further stratified by selecting from each such region one PCC sponsored by the Conservative party; one sponsored by the Labour party, and one independent PCC (i.e. without affiliation to a formally-recognised political party). At the same time, care was taken in the selection process to ensure a reasonable cross-section of urban and rural of police force areas (the final sample comprising PCCs for two metropolitan force areas; four for more mixed urban/rural force areas; and three for force areas that were more rural in character).

While no strong claims are made about the overall representativeness of this sample, or indeed, of the pattern of responses derived from it[2], the key findings and general messages at least are probably not untypical of the wider picture across the country. The interviews were conducted (by the author) on a one-to-one basis and in a semi-structured format[3] between July and October 2013 (i.e. between 8 and 12 months after the elections). In preparation for the interviews, a range of documentary information published on each PCC's website was also reviewed (including Annual Reports, Police and Crime Plans, budgetary and commissioning reports, policy statements, minutes of meetings, formal decisions, blogs, and other such communications).

Accountability to the Public

Probably the most significant finding from the nine interviews concerned the large commitment of time and effort that, since the elections, each PCC had been devoting to building their profiles with the public and local communities. Perhaps, in part, a reaction to the very poor turnout at the polls and the very low level of public understanding of the new role, all nine PCCs had made it their first priority to pursue as many opportunities as possible for public engagement and for building relationships with local institutions and groups across their areas as well as with officers and staff at each of the police stations.

Interestingly, one of the nine who had previously served as a member of the (former) police authority for the area, suggested that *'police authorities hadn't thought of themselves as having a public profile'*—a viewpoint that, if fair, would possibly go some way towards accounting for the very low level of public awareness of their existence. Yet within a matter of days of taking office, all nine PCCs had begun a circuit of public appearances, making presentations and answering questions at public meetings, arranging regular 'surgeries' in local communities, and 'pitching up' in market squares on Saturday mornings to meet shoppers, just as they had done during their election campaigns. Each had also begun a round of attendances at county, district and parish/town council meetings and had accepted a variety of invi-

---

[2] For example, the sample did not include a PCC who had previously served as a police officer, although nationally, about 1 in 5 of the 41 who were elected had done so. Just two of the nine PCCs were female while, as far as ethnicity was concerned, all were white.

[3] In three of the nine cases, a senior assistant to the commissioner was also present for the interview. To protect and respect confidentiality, the nine PCCs and their areas are cited in this chapter simply as numbers (1–9 respectively).

tations to speak at meetings of other community bodies such as Women's Institutes, Rotary, and Volunteer Centres.

They were also spending much time visiting different policing and criminal justice-related projects, including many community-based and volunteer-run initiatives undertaking community safety work or supporting criminal justice, for example, victim support groups, domestic abuse projects, drug-treatment centres and various offender management projects. Indeed, all nine indicated spending at least a day per week away from their offices meeting community-based, staff and volunteers involved in criminal justice-related project work of one kind or another or addressing open meetings, community councils and the like. Many of their evenings were also taken up with speaking engagements and each was frequently writing articles for local magazines, community newsletters and bulletins. All were also making extensive use of social media—with near daily tweets and regular blogs on policing and crime issues arising from their work.

Clearly, then, the new PCCs have, without exception prioritised their relationships with their local public(s) and sought to provide a significantly more outward-facing governance profile than had been the case with police authorities. Moreover, and no doubt a consequence of such profile-raising efforts, each confirmed having seen the volume of direct communications from members of the public (via email, letter or phone calls) increase significantly. One commented that *"PCCs are set to become some of the most recognised public leaders in the country—more so than most local councillors and many members of parliament"*, while another pointed out that *"the police themselves are amazed at what this is all producing by way of complaints from public."*

Several interviewees also emphasised the importance they attached to hearing from all sections of the community, not just those who had made contact to complain about something or who had spoken up at a public meeting or other event. One, for example, talked at length about actively seeking out the perspectives of those who were perhaps unlikely to attend such meetings or to initiate contact— *"the quiet ones; the NEETs, ethnic groups and others below the radar"*. And such pro-activity certainly suggested a further positive dimension to the *"listening and learning"* approach to which all nine referred. Also highlighted was the contact with front-line policing teams; each having already visited, or being in the process of visiting, every police station within their areas, and from which they similarly indicated gaining highly valuable learning, not least about the issues and problems of most concern locally. *"Only by listening and talking to front-line police and the public do you get a sense of whether or not resources are being satisfactorily deployed within the Force…being out and about and listening is how you learn about how the force is working"*. As another summed the discussion up, *"…listening is what this job is all about—people say things to you in the street that they wouldn't say to you in a booked appointment or if they were come into the building"*.

Evidently, then, 'listening and learning', has clearly formed a highly significant dimension of PCC work. And while this of course would not by itself necessarily amount to strong accountability, it would at least form a key element of such a process. Indeed, in so far as all the interviewees talked about the lively exchanges in which they were frequently engaged in public meetings, it seemed that the twin processes of 'giving account' and 'being held to account' were, indeed, very much a part of this on-going public engagement process.

Accountability to the Police and Crime Panels

As indicated, the same legislation instituting PCCs also introduced Police and Crime Panels to undertake a scrutiny role and hold commissioners to account on behalf of the public. Indeed, such Panels were established to provide an on-going check on the work of the PCC between elections when the voting public would have their say on the office-holder's performance, and as a means to address the 'information asymmetry problem' of the principal-agent relationship between the public and the PCC.

That said, the legitimate roles of the Police and Crime Panel are quite tightly defined in the relevant statutes and relate particularly to scrutinising the annual budget, approval of the Police and Crime Plan (a 5-year strategy document that each PCC is required to prepare and publish) and approval of the appointment of the chief constable. Such scrutiny roles are also balanced by a more general 'supportive' role that, as Lister (2014. p. 24) has pointed out *"must be exercised with a view to supporting the effective exercise of the functions of the police and crime commissioner"*. This, as Lister has also suggested, implies some tension at the heart of the legislation, although, to be fair, this was also inherent in the role (and behaviour) of the former police authorities which similarly could be understood as 'critical friends' (in their case to the chief constable). But whereas the former police authorities had a clear oversight and scrutiny role in relation to policing performance, the focus of the Police and Crime Panels is much more narrowly drawn in relation to the work of the PCC, who, in turn, is soley responsible for holding the chief constable to account.

From the interviews the evidence as to the nature of accountability at work here seemed quite mixed. All nine acknowledged the difficulties that both the limited statutory powers and the tight (Government-imposed) timetable had created in the first year for panel members in their consideration of the budgets and the Police and Crime Plans and more generally in the process of holding to account. Two PCCs specifically commented on the shift they had observed in the outlook of their panels—from initial scepticism and negativity to becoming generally supportive once they had heard the Commissioner's explanations and had understood better the thinking behind the choices and decisions. Two others observed that panel members with previous experience on their respective police authorities had seemed to struggle to come to terms with their new role as 'scrutineers' of the Commissioner's (personally-taken) decisions. Others again recognised the difficulties in this regard for panels of part-time councillors (from across the area) in scrutinising the decisions of a full-time PCC (and with considerably greater officer support and informational resources to call upon)—in other words, the 'principal-agent' problem of 'information asymmetry'.

Even so, three PCCs were quite critical of the quality of scrutiny offered by their panels; one describing the process as "*a bit tokenistic*", another as "*without real teeth*" and "*not very dynamic*", and a third, more bluntly still, as "*a wholly inadequate way of holding you to account*". Indeed, none felt the holding to account process to have been particularly onerous, and none had been asked by their Panels to provide additional information or to consider particular actions (as the statutes allow). On the contrary, in three instances, it had been the PCCs who had taken the initiative and invited the panels to assist them by undertaking additional work—of a supportive nature. In one instance, the panel had been in two minds about whether or not to accept such an invitation although in the other two instances, there had been willingness to assist and become more actively engaged with their PCCs as a result.

It would have been helpful in this context to have been able to compare the perspectives of PCCs on the accountability provided by Police and Crime Panels with those of panellists themselves, though to do so was beyond the scope of the particular research project. But it was interesting that, from the commissioners' viewpoints at least, the contribution of the panels was seen very much along the lines that Lister (2014) had predicted—with a somewhat uneasy tension between the respective roles of providing scrutiny on the one hand and support on the other, or what Coulson and Whiteman (2012) have summarised as a 'critical friend' relationship. Partly, it was suggested by one PCC, the difficulty here was compounded by the tendency in many areas for the constituent local authorities to prefer to nominate a senior political leader as their representative on the panel (in most instances, the council leader or a cabinet member for community safety) rather than a councillor with particular aptitude for scrutiny work and with the analytical skills by which to hold executive personnel to account. Worse, as pointed out by one PCC, because of diary congestion for many such senior political leaders, substitutes were often asked to attend the meetings in place of the official nominees with consequential discontinuity effects for the membership of the panels.

Accountability to Central Government

A third accountability relationship for PCCs, also enshrined in legislation, and which again the PCC is in an 'agent' role, is in relation to central government, particularly regarding national strategic policing requirements. Besides this particular statutory responsibility on PCCs to support national policing needs, for example, in relation to serious organised crime, terrorism, cyber-crime and other criminal activity that exceeds local territorial boundaries, however, is a wider issue about the extent of influence by the Home Office and Home Secretary upon PCC discretion. From the outset with PCCs, this was always likely to be potentially significant issue, not just because of the strongly centralist culture that had long characterised the Home Office as a department of state, but also because of the high political stakes for the Coalition Government in relation to the launch of the new PCC governance model.

Particularly in light of the plethora of uncomfortable media headlines around the time of the first elections, it would have been surprising, indeed, had the inevitable anxieties in and around Whitehall and Westminster not prompted at least consideration of a more interventionist approach to stabilise matters. But then, as indicated, the PCC model had also been devised, promoted and launched within the context of the Coalition Government's policy commitment towards 'new localism' (Lowndes and Pratchett 2012). Indeed, the model had itself been much cited by ministers as a leading exemplar of the commitment to localism.

Despite such a context, the clear feedback from the nine PCCs who were interviewed was that they had each been left largely to get on with their roles at local level in the manner they individually considered most appropriate, and with minimal interference or imposition from the Home Office. Although recognising their obligations in support of the national 'strategic policing requirement', none saw this as presenting contentious pressures for them, or creating particular conflicts with their own commitments and priorities. On the contrary, all nine commented positively on the constructive balance they felt the Home Office had struck between providing support, if and when requested (including good access to the Home Secretary in person), and allowing each to go about their role in their own way, for example, organising and staffing their offices, determining their own policing priorities, and establishing working relations with chief constables as they felt most fitting.

Interestingly, however, several PCCs contrasted this state of affairs in relation to the Home Office—the lead department of government for policing—with what they saw as a very different stance of the other key department of state with which they had interactions—the Ministry of Justice. Of particular concern to PCCs at the time of the interviews in this respect was the Ministry's decision to implement its new commissioning framework for probation services not on the well-established territorial structure of local criminal justice (i.e. the 41 PCC areas) but instead on the basis of 21 regions. Two PCCs also aired concerns at the possible prospect of their legitimate discretion being compromised in future if HM Inspectorate of Constabulary reviews and reports were to cover strategic governance issues as well as operational policing matters.

Accountability to Political Sponsors

A fourth accountability relationship affecting many PCCs applies to those who stood for election as candidates for a particular political party. Again, this casts the PCC in an 'agent' relationship to the sponsoring political party (as 'principal') and it was of interest to examine to what extent this imposed constraints and pressures upon the office-holders' decision-making and scope for action in practice—the issue of the potential introduction of partisan politics into policing being a key criticism of the model when first announced. In fact in the elections in 2012 some 138 candidates were sponsored by one or other of the political parties while a further 54 (less than 1 in 4) stood as 'independents' (i.e. without affiliation to a political party).

Of the 41 who were elected to office, 29 were sponsored by a political party (16 by the Conservative party and 13 by the Labour party), while the other 12 (nearly 1 in 3) were 'independents'. As Lister and Rowe (2015) have suggested, this relatively strong showing by the 'independent' candidates in the ballot rather suggested that many voters also shared the concern about potential politicisation of policing (and indeed most of the 'independent' candidates had focused on this concern as part of their own election campaigns).

That said, the interviews with the sample of PCCs (three Conservative, three Labour and three Independents) revealed little clear evidence to support such concerns in practice. Perhaps unsurprisingly, all three Conservative PCCs and all three Labour PCCs (like their three independent counterparts) spoke of the importance they attached to serving all interests within their areas, and for pursuing priorities for policing that would be reflective of the needs and aspirations of all its communities. Indeed, as one (Conservative party-sponsored) PCC pointed out: "*a clear message from the [election] campaign was that the public don't want politics in policing—so the rosettes are off*".

On the other hand the interviews did reveal some interesting differences between the PCCs with regard to their overarching perspectives, outlooks and ambitions for their roles, and which could perhaps be understood in macro-political terms. The three Conservative PCCs, for instance, each conveyed a strong managerialist polity in expressing their determination to improve efficiency and value for money in policing. They also spoke at length about their ambitions to '*get upstream*' by investing more strongly in crime prevention and in better support for families where there were risks of anti-social behaviour or involvement in crime. While such ambitions were probably shared by all the other PCCs, it was noteworthy that the three Labour PCCs talked much more about local issues in their areas; about some of the casework arising from their surgeries, and about their prioritisation of particular crime and anti-social behaviour problems in particular neighbourhoods or afflicting particular social groups. In short, here seemed to be a rather different polity from that of their Conservative counterparts—one much more about '*problem-solving*' in the shorter-term.

Probably such contrasting polities would also reflect differences of geography—and particularly the socio-economic and criminogenic contrasts between the more suburban/rural police areas on the one hand (which had elected Conservative and Independent PCCs), and the more densely populated urban/metropolitan areas on the other (which had elected Labour candidates). At the same time, however, the respective career backgrounds of the PCCs seemed also to be a relevant factor here. It was noteworthy, for example, that the three Labour PCCs had each been active in politics for significant periods of their careers, and indeed, within much the same geographical area. All had served as councillors, and two had gravitated to national level as MPs for their local constituencies. Perhaps, then, the commitment they each articulated towards problem-solving on behalf of communities, groups and individuals had its roots in their previous experience as constituency and ward-level politicians.

In similar vein, those PCCs with background experience in the judiciary tended to articulate a particularly strong concern for issues of fairness and equity. One who had served as a magistrate, for instance, talked of concerns about the force's 'stop and search' policies and practices and spoke of the challenges in communicating with hard-to-reach groups and minorities. Another raised the subject of domestic and sexual abuse and violence and talked about prioritising responses to this in their Police and Crime Plan. A third, with a judicial experience in the Crown Court, spoke of the potential of restorative justice approaches in dealing with offenders of petty crime.

Meanwhile, it was noteworthy that all three Conservative PCCs not only had a business management background, but had also, more recently, all served in political leadership roles within their (Conservative-controlled) local authorities (settings where the strategic objectives of achieving better value for money through more integrated public service provision have been particularly strongly emphasised in the past few years). Two of the three such Conservative PCCs, talked of what they felt to be a stark contrast between the limited inter-agency collaboration and co-ordination within policing and criminal justice on the one hand and the more integrative developments now taking place in the local authorities with which they were familiar. *"The police talk endlessly about strategy but are not good at it. Most of their work is about meeting deadlines in minutes and hours, and they struggle to lift their sights towards the longer term"*, suggested one of them, while the other expressed particular frustration at what he saw as the huge scope for achieving greater efficiency through more neighbouring forces and other agencies working more closely together with other local public service providers and pooled budgets *"to prevent crime rather than having to react to it afterwards"*. Both spoke critically of what they regarded to be outdated practices in their police forces and highlighted some of the traditions that they felt to be *'self-serving'*. One commented that he *"hadn't prepared [myself] for the shambolic state of the business side of policing—not policing itself—but the systems and processes by which it is managed"*.

That said, more complex differences between the three groups (Conservative, Labour and Independent PCCs) were highlighted in an analysis of the priorities formally adopted by each of the nine PCCs in their Police and Crime Plans. In this respect, as can be seen in Table 9.1, beyond the fact that the three Labour-sponsored PCCs had each proposed a significantly larger number of priorities than those of either their Conservative or Independent counterparts (an average of 9 compared with one of less than 4 per PCC), there appeared little obvious group-based patterning in the chosen priorities Indeed, rather than differences, the two most notable features from the analysis seemed to be, on the one hand, the degree of commonality across the three groups and, on the other, the shared commitment to very generalised pledges such as: 'reducing and preventing crime', 'protecting the public', 'customer care', and 'better value for money'.

Table 9.1 Police and crime plan priorities of the nine PCCs

Sample of PCCs Priority	Labour-sponsored			Conservative-sponsored			Independent		
	1	2	3	4	5	6	7	8	9
Reducing and preventing crime (esp burglary)	X	X	X			X	X	X	X
Protecting people		X	X			X		X	
Customer care/quality of service	X	X			X			X	
Better value for money		X			X				X
Victims at the heart of criminal justice				X		X	X		
Violence against women (domestic violence)	X					X	X		
Making the public feel safer	X	X							X
Improving public confidence		X		X					
Effective partnerships	X	X							
Anti-social behaviour	X						X		
Youth offending and youth justice	X								
Restorative justice	X								
Working with the CJS	X								
Supporting stronger communities		X							
Action against hate crime			X						
Police standards and social responsibility		X							
Making offenders pay (for police services)					X				
Effective contribution to national policing		X							
Developing local identity		X							
Tackling serious and organised crime			X						
Providing visible neighbourhood policing			X						
Early interventions to tackle roots of crime				X					
Road safety	X								
Tackling on-line crime (including child abuse)	X								
A well-led and skilled workforce								X	

Holding the Chief Constable to Account

Thus far the focus has been on four accountability relationships in which PCCs could be understood as the 'agent'—respectively to the public and voters, to the police and crime panels, to the Home Office/central government, and to political sponsors. But in the relationship with the chief constable, as indicated earlier, the PCC acts as the 'principal' and faces the classic Principal-Agent problem of being formally in charge but with less knowledge of the subject in question than the 'agent' (in this case, the chief constable) who will undertake the work. So how can the PCC be sure that the police will do as expected of them, and how might the chief constable and the force be held to account? In fact the problem in the PCC context is further complicated by the 'operational independence' that is afforded in statute to the chief constable and which denies the PCC authority to provide directions on matters of day-to-day policing work. Moreover, this is a complication that is not made any easier by the lack of formal guidance from the Home Office on what exactly constitutes 'operational' responsibility (Lister 2014).

The potential for tension in the PCC-chief constable relationship was recognised from the outset when several senior police officers were outspoken in their criticism of the model and then when a number retired early or failed to have their contracts renewed. On the other hand, it should be said that, in the context of accountability, tension between PCC and chief constable could of course be positive in ensuring that the agent performs as the principal would wish, while a working relationship that is too close and comfortable in nature could well be problematical if it masks under-performance.

Among the nine interviewees there was certainly keen awareness of the significance of the less-than-clearly-defined 'boundary line' between their own more strategic area of responsibility and that for operational policing of their chief constable. Indeed, from the comments and examples proffered it seemed that boundary line had been (gently) 'tested' on more than one occasion during the course of the first year. Mostly, however, relationships with chief constables were described in positive terms, with very few on-going disagreements highlighted over division of responsibilities. Two of the nine had in fact made their own new chief constable appointment since the election following the resignation or non-reappointment of a predecessor, so were (unsurprisingly) content with the relationship. Another also described their working relationship as '*good*', but emphasised the importance of the '*keeping of distance*' and '*retaining a certain formality*'. For two others again, '*very positive working relationships*' were explained as having resulted from a working relationship at local level that had preceded the elections. Meanwhile, another, who similarly knew the chief well from having served on the former police authority, indicated having had some differences of opinion on a number of key strategic issues, and described the position somewhat diplomatically as '*an appropriate working relationship*'.

In the case of the other three commissioners, two described their relationships with their chief constables as '*good*' although, in both instances, adding that it was still '*early days*'; both regarding it as '*an evolving relationship*' with '*learning taking place on both sides as to the other's expectations*'. Meanwhile, in the other instance, an initially '*difficult relationship*' had, after several fraught months, begun to resolve itself to the extent that the chief constable had been awarded a new contract for a further term.

All nine interviewees reported holding regular formal meetings with their chief constables for the purpose of 'holding to account' (and with official minutes taken of such meetings). In most instances such meetings were held either weekly or fortnightly, though in one case, it was twice weekly and in another, every six weeks (having initially been monthly). In each case, however, it was emphasised that interactions with the chief constable of a less formal nature took place on a near daily basis, either face-to-face or by telephone, and usually to discuss a particular issue that had arisen, or in the form of a briefing on a new development.

Such patterns of contact would undoubtedly be much facilitated by the choice made by six of the PCCs to establish their offices within the confines of police headquarters. However, particularly in light of all the comments about the importance of public profile and accountability to local people, it was perhaps a little surprising that most had prioritised proximity to the chief constable and senior officers over more publicly accessible locations (without the high levels of security control for visitors that characterise most police headquarters). But in each case, the reason for the decision was explained in terms of saving office costs by making use of available (and free) police accommodation. In fact, of the three PCCs who had located themselves away from their force headquarters, two had actually chosen to occupy part of a local police station (in one case a former one) within their areas, so again making use of available space. The third was occupying city centre accommodation that had previously provided the headquarters of the former police authority (although the PCC indicated a desire to sell the building and relocate to less expensive premises in a more centrally-positioned location within the police area as a whole).

Conclusions

In this chapter the aim has been to take stock of the impacts of the introduction of police and crime commissioners particularly with regard to the different accountability relationships involved, doing so on the basis of a series of interviews with PCCs around the country. Above all the interviews highlighted the extent to which office holders have worked at building relationships with their local public and so fostering an on-going process of public accountability. In contrast, the interviews found that the three other accountability relationships in which the PCC was involved as 'agent' were much less significant in practice. The Police and Crime Panels, in the first year at least, were generally playing a fairly marginal role in holding the commissioners to account; the Home Office had resisted the centre's usual controlling and standardising temptations and, for the most part, had left PCCs to develop the role as they individually felt best; and the political party sponsors were similarly, to date at least, unimportant in directing or pressuring 'their' PCCs. Meanwhile, with regard to the converse accountability relationships—those in which the PCC was 'principal' (to the chief constable, as 'agent') the interviews highlighted generally effective working relationships, with clear evidence of effective 'holding to account', and with signs of greater governance impact and influence on policing priorities and practices than had previously been the case under police authorities.

In identifying and highlighting the efforts of PCCs to build relationships and foster accountability with the public, it should of course be recognised that, in part at least such efforts might well be motivated by self-interest to ensure future re-electoral success. Even so, however, it was clear that each PCC was also driven by desire to acquire good personal understanding of public expectations about policing and crime reduction and to ensure that such understandings could be reflected in their own prioritisations of policing resources and in their approach to the role more generally. In this sense the interest in listening to the public and 'taking [such viewpoint] into account', could be understood as Ashworth and Skelcher (2005) have argued, as a key step in building accountability. And such listening and 'taking into account' was amply illustrated within the Police and Crime Plans published by PCCs in March 2013; some exemplary phrases of which are reproduced below in Table 9.2.

It is, as Newburn (2013) has suggested, too early yet to reach firm conclusions about the impacts of the new model of police governance through PCCs. But the

Table 9.2 Statements from the Police and Crime Plans of the nine sampled PCCs

"I will take an analytic, evidence-based approach to reducing crime and disorder and for creating healthy safe communities. It will be based on a sound foundation of understanding and engaging with the public…" (PCC 1)

"I am keen that this plan captures the voice of the public on how priorities are developed and set…" (PCC 2)

"In determining my priorities I have listened to the views that the public have expressed through engagement events and feedback questionnaires. I have also spoken to partner agencies, such as community safety partnerships and the Criminal Justice Board, as well as considering the professional judgement of the Chief Constable." (PCC 3)

"The new agenda signals more focus and investment to prevent crime or anti-social behaviour before it happens, with the police, local authorities and other agencies joining up better to tackle what causes crime, not just the effects of it…I also want everyone involved to be honest and brave by stopping things that haven't worked in the past, or don't join up properly, in favour of starting things that do." (PCC4)

"In every aspect of this plan I set out what I want to see from the police, from partner organisations and, critically, from the public." (PCC 5)

"My vision of safer neighbourhoods, improved levels of public confidence, crime reduction, public protection and more responsive victim services can only become a reality if I can continue to harness the energy and enthusiasm of the public to become a key part of the solution." (PCC 6)

"This plan sets out our Police and Crime priorities for 2013–2017 which are based on the issues you have raised. You have told me that your concerns are anti-social behaviour, burglary and domestic and sexual violence. I will ensure that wherever you live—rural, suburban, town or city—your police will work with you and have the flexibility to deliver these priorities." (PCC 7)

"Although the chief constable and his officers are a primary audience for the Plan, my aim is to place stakeholders, users of the service, and beneficiaries at the heart of it. My intention is that it will provide the public, including partner agencies and victims of crim, a clear understanding of what they can expect from the police service and the Commissioner…" (PCC 8)

"I have listened to your experiences, concerns, and suggestions; I have met hundreds of you face-to-face and corresponded with hundreds more. It's a continuing and essential dialogue that means you help to decide where money and manpower can do most good. So in a very real sense, this is your Police and Crime Plan. You are my co-authors because you know your communities better than anyone else. And together we can ensure that tax-payers' money—YOUR money—is spent where it can genuinely benefit the public." (PCC 9) story so far seems to be of police governance in England and Wales becoming more visible, more consultative and, by implication, more publicly accountable too.

References

Ashworth, R., & Skelcher, C. (2005). Meta-evaluation of the local government modernisation agenda: Progress report on accountability in local government.

Bandyopadhyay, S. (2013). Crime policy in an era of Austerity. *Police Journal, 86*(2), 102–115.

Bertelli, A. M. (2012). *The political economy of public sector governance.* Cambridge New York: Cambridge University Press.

Besley, T. (2006). *Principled agents? The political economy of good government.* Oxford: Oxford University Press.

Bovaird, T., Briggs, I., & Willis, M. (2013). Strategic commissioning in the UK: Service improvement cycle or just going round in circles? *Local Government Studies, 40*(1), 23–36.

Coulson, A., & Whiteman, P. (2012). Holding politicians to account? Overview and scrutiny in English local government. *Public Money and Management, 32*(3), 185–192.

Ferris, J. M., & Graddy, E. A. (1998). A contractual framework for new public management theory. *International Public Management Journal, 16*(1), 225–240.

Home Office. (2008). From the neighbourhood to the national: Policing our communities together, White paper Cm 7448,The Stationery Office: London.

H M Government (2010). The Coalition: Our Programme for Government, London: Cabinet Office.

Independent Police Commission. (2013). Policing for a better Britain: Report of the independent police commission, 25th-November-2013.

Knott, J. H., & Miller, G. J. (2006). Social welfare, corruption and credibility: Public management's role in economic development. *Public Management Review, 8*(2), 227–252.

Laville, S. (2013). Court overturns 'irrational' decision to suspend Lincolnshire chief constable. *The Guardian.*

Lister, S. (2014). Scrutinising the role of the police and crime panel in the new era of police governance in England and Wales. *Safer Communities, 13*(1), 22–31.

Lister, S., & Rowe, M. (2015). Electing police and crime commissioners in England and Wales: Prospecting for the democratisation of policing. *Policing and Society, 1*, 1–20.

Lowndes, V., & Pratchett, L. (2012). Local governance under the coalition government: Austerity, localism and the big society. *Local Government Studies, 38*(1), 21–40.

Mayston, D. (1993). Principal, agents, and the economics of accountability in the new public sector. *Accounting, Auditing & Accountability Journal, 6*, 68–96.

Newburn, T. (2013). The Stevens report, British politics and policy at LSE, Blog November 2013, London: London School of Economics; http://eprints.lse.ac.uk/54786/.

Raine, J. W. (2014). Electocracy with accountabilities? The novel governance model of police and crime commissioners. In S. Lister & M. Rowe (Eds.), *Policing and accountability.* London: Routledge.

Raine, J. W., & Keasey, P. (2012). From police authorities to police and crime commissioners: Might policing become more publicly accountable? *International Journal of Emergency Services, 1*(2), 122–134.

Waterman, R. W., & Meier, K. J. (1998). Principal-agent models: An expansion? *Journal of Public Administration Research & Theory, 8*, 173.

Wood, D., & Waterman, R. (1994). *Bureaucratic dynamics: The role of bureaucracy in a democracy.* Oxford: Westview Press.

John W. Raine BA PhD is Professor of Management in Criminal Justice at the University of Birmingham, U.K. His research interests embrace governance, policy and management issues across the criminal justice sector, but particularly in policing, the courts, offender management and victim support work. As well as being a leading researcher and author in such fields, John also has strong research interests in relation to local authority regulation and enforcement. He frequently acts as a consultant to both national government and to local agencies and has served as a member of the Criminal Justice Council of England and Wales since its establishment in 2002.

Chapter 10
Police Management and Workforce Reform in a Period of Austerity

Barry Loveday

Introduction

Since the arrival of the Coalition Government in 2010 the police have been subject to a degree of reform almost unexampled since the restructuring of the police service following the Police Act of 1964 and subsequent police mergers. However in contrast to the earlier reforms which ultimately created much bigger and semi- autonomous police forces the current reform programme has proved to be much more intrusive. Indeed it has explicitly set out to bring the police service much closer to the community it serves and also to make it much more responsive to local needs and local priorities.

This significant change in relationship has been led by the creation of local Police and Crime Commissioners (PCCs) for each police force area. Introduced by way of the Police Reform and Social Responsibility Act 2011, PCCs are both directly elected and able to exercise wide powers in relation to the appointment and dismissal of chief officers. Having responsibility for the budget and also for the local police and crime plan the PCC is now able to exercise a considerable influence over policing priorities in the local area.

PCCs

This is made manifest by the fact that while PCCs have no desire to challenge the operational independence of the police they are committed to establishing a clear principal and agent relationship between PCC and Chief Officer, where the chief

B. Loveday (✉)
University of Portsmouth, Portsmouth, UK
e-mail: barry.loveday@port.ac.uk

© Springer International Publishing Switzerland 2015
P. Wankhade, D. Weir (eds.), *Police Services,* DOI 10.1007/978-3-319-16568-4_10

officer as agent is made directly accountable to the PCC. This in itself is a remarkable reversal of roles which pertained between chief officers and police authorities where the latter appeared to be little more than the agent of the chief constable. This change in relationship has of course proved very difficult for a number of chief officers to accept and has explained the undoubted tensions that have arisen within some police areas between chief officers and their PCCs (Loveday 2013; Policy Exchange 2013).

However the reform of police governance has proved to be not the only substantive change demanded of the police by the Coalition government. Thus for the first time in decades the police service has also had to share the burden of severe spending cuts with other public services. The decision to impose a 20% cut in police spending has been a wake- up call to a public service long protected from cuts and where over the past three decades spending has ballooned to just over £ 8 billion a year (Home Office 2014). The decision to implement spending cuts while defended at the time by reference to the need for austerity may also have reflected a growing recognition that much of police spending might not provide value for money and had little impact on the crime rate either (Loveday 2008b; Policy Exchange 2012).

The Winsor Report 2012

Yet the most challenging feature of the new period of austerity has proved to be the quite radical conclusions of the Winsor Report which was to recommend a wide range of reform to police pay and conditions which it claimed were designed 'for a different era' (Winsor 2012, p. 11). Among a range of reform proposals the recommendation to in effect end overtime pay and all special payments while also cutting the starting pay of new recruits served to concentrate the minds of all police associations but particularly the Police Federation, traditionally viewed as the most powerful 'voice of the police service'.

The Winsor report represented a frontal attack on all the gains that the Police Federation had achieved over 30 years. This was best evidenced in the additional recommendation made by Winsor that chief officers for the very first time be given the power of compulsory severance of sworn officers where that was deemed necessary. This would allow chief officers to more effectively manage their police forces while enabling them to 'change their workforce mix or structure' and a workforce flexibility that was now required (Winsor 2012, p. 291). For Winsor the primary drivers for reform revolved around ensuring the police service provided 'more for less'. As was argued within the Report:

> For too long, police forces have enjoyed unpressurised financial settlements. This state of affairs has in too many respects engendered practices of waste and inefficiency. This must change. It is almost inevitable that the economic condition of the country will maintain or intensify the need for improved performance against reducing budgets. (Winsor 2012, p. 13)

The Winsor recommendations represent a sea- change in the approach to police funding and management. Traditionally successive Governments have either sought to protect but usually increase police spending. This was usually based on a number of factors but not least an untested assumption that increasing police establishment would impact on crime rates. Perhaps as significant increased spending on police officers publicly demonstrated that successive Governments were 'tough on crime' and where elements of the popular press identified spending on police numbers as an indicator of government commitment to this objective (Loveday 2013, p. 100). This was to be perhaps best demonstrated with New Labour's explicit commitment to increasing police establishment by ring-fencing spending on additional police numbers. Unfortunately (and as in the past), little was required by Government thereafter for police forces to demonstrate the extent to which either increased spending or establishment had influenced either the crime rate or perceptions of personal safety (fear of crime). This problem was to be further complicated by the Blair government's renewed commitment to performance management and the introduction of wide ranging performance targets for police forces. The inevitable pressure to adopt gaming strategies in response to this made any realistic measurement of police effectiveness much more difficult to undertake (Loveday 2006). Moreover as recent revelations concerning the 'massaging' of police recording of crime demonstrate, traditional measures of effectiveness will now need to be readdressed (Ford 2013).

Power of Compulsory Severance

Yet the full implications of the Winsor report may have proved too difficult a challenge for even the current Home Secretary. While adopting a strong not to say an intransigent position on police pay cuts not least in face of overt and aggressive opposition at successive annual Police Federation Conferences (traditionally the reputational graveyard of successive Home Secretaries) the important decision concerning the issue of police severance appears to have eluded her. Thus the ratification by the Home Secretary of the Police Arbitration Tribunal's ruling against compulsory severance may mark the high watermark of police reform. While the Home Secretary has also stated that it 'remained a reform the government and the police should continue to consider' it is evident that it will not be the current Coalition government that will undertake this reform (Martis 2014).

The failure to implement the Winsor recommendation of compulsory severance could prove a significant challenge to improving the internal management of the police service and therefore its performance. As it currently stands the inability of chief officers to make flexible use of their workforce acts a major impediment to improved efficiency. The situation has been highlighted both within the Winsor Report and also by earlier evidence from a number of workforce modernisation 'demonstration sites' where flexible employment arrangements have been found to be one important way of improving police efficiency (Loveday 2008a). As Winsor notes currently police forces are made up of two 'substantially different workforces: police officers who are not employees and police staff who are' (Winsor 2012, p. 295).

While police managers have the same management powers as do other employers in relation to civilian staff (voluntary severance, early retirement and compulsory redundancy) this does not extend to police officers. As is noted currently it is not possible for a police force to require a police officer with less than 30 years service to resign on the grounds of efficiency. The result is that the grounds on which a police officer can be required to leave the police service are very limited and therefore 'provide very little flexibility to manage the officer workforce to meet future needs'. As a result the only way police managers can reduce police numbers is by suspending recruitment to reduce police officer numbers or reducing establishment through natural wastage (Winsor 2012, p. 295). Other than providing a level of job protection that does not obtain anywhere else in the public service the inability to manage police officer numbers means that the current status of police officers creates the perverse effect of undermining overall police efficiency and effectiveness.

This is because, as has been demonstrated vividly in the recent programme of police budget cuts, police managers will exercise powers of compulsory severance over civilian staff to achieve the spending reductions requested 'as it is easier to cut staff posts' (HMIC 2012, p. 24). One consequence of this can be the removal of staff who may often have crucial roles within the police force and the withdrawal of police officers from operational duties to take on the duties previously undertaken by civilian staff. As will be argued later, the issue of police jobs for life could prove to be the litmus test of any attempt to modernise policing and introduce effective management within the police service. It is however also seen, unsurprisingly as a litmus test by the Police Federation which is determined to retain this remarkable level of job protection both as a defence of their members but also of the self espoused 'independence of the office of constable' (Martis 2014).

Internal Management Change-Outsourcing

Following on from the decision taken by both Cleveland Police and Avon and Somerset Constabulary to sign up to 10 year contracts with private suppliers to provide support services, this option has been explored by a number of other police forces. The decision to consider outsourcing has been universally linked to the 20% cuts in police budgets imposed under the Comprehensive Spending Review (CSR) which was to initiate a major programme of cuts across the public sector. What marked out the 2010 CSR was the decision to extend this process to the police service and bring to an end what had been an uninterrupted period of spending increases spread over three decades (Loveday 2013).

It may also be the case that Ministers within the Cabinet Office are encouraging police forces to consider the potential savings which outsourcing may offer. In this capacity Francis Maude has for example sought to extend the role of private suppliers within public sector services. This commitment remains in place even where dubious business practices have proved to characterise the activities of at least one major supplier. The appointment, from the private sector, of a 'crown representative' to oversee the conduct of one major contractor (G4S) is deemed to provide, within the government anyway, sufficient reassurance for the future (Muir 2014).

Yet irrespective of potential ethical issues that might arise as a consequence of business practices among private contractors the evident appeal of outsourcing remains clear. This is because the saving achieved through outsourcing can be expected to roughly match the budget cuts imposed on police forces as a consequence of the 2010 CSA. By embracing private sector support, police chiefs are aware that savings from back office functions can help maintain visible policing in the force area. There are, however, potential costs to this development which need to be considered and which in some police areas have clearly influenced the decision not to go forward with this initiative.

Thus in both Surrey and West Midlands earlier interest in outsourcing has not survived the arrival of Police and Crime Commissioners where as in West Midlands the PCC was to indicate his complete opposition early on (BBC West Midlands 2012). Nor have the earlier aspirations of contractors to undertake the support role for three East Midland forces to be realised as the PCCs for Hertfordshire, Bedfordshire and Cambridgeshire discontinued negotiations with the contractor-G4S-as the contract was deemed 'unsuitable for the unique position of the three forces' (Cockerell 2014). This is not however likely to mean that further investigation of outsourcing for these forces will not be undertaken. It is evident that the PCC for Hertfordshire is ready to negotiate with other market providers and has stated that he believes 'that substantial elements of policing support services will be best delivered by the private sector and will ensure that this option is immediately explored' (Cockerell 2014).

Just how significant the impact of outsourcing can prove to be for the future profile of an individual police force is very clearly demonstrated with the example of Lincolnshire Police whose police authority was to formalise the contract in 2011. Under the contract, worth in excess of £ 200 millions, G4S has taken responsibility for the Police Custody and Identification Unit; Force control room; Town Enquiry officers; Crime Management Bureau; Central Ticket office and Collisions Unit; Criminal Justice Unit; Firearms Licensing and Resource Management Unit. G4S now also provides 'business support' to Lincolnshire Police Human Resources Services; HR Learning and development; Assets and Facilities Management (including Fleet management); Finance and Procurement and Support Services. While this allowed the force 'space to begin to bridge the financial gap' created by the CSR and create the 'leanest police force in Britain' it also meant that for the foreseeable future the force had relinquished control of a major element of its support service infrastructure (Lincolnshire Police Authority 2011). Given the length of the contract this responsibility would be unlikely to ever return to the police force (Loveday 2013).

Savings and Costs of Outsourcing

It is immediately apparent that major savings to the police force can be assured initially with the removal of all sworn police officers from back office duties. National pay agreements and pay scales have of course made police officers highly expensive and significantly better paid than any other emergency service (Loveday 2013). In Cleveland the short term savings were to follow on from the entire removal of 200 warranted offices from back room functions. Nor given their current cost are they ever likely to return to these duties under outsourcing arrangements. In Lincolnshire cost savings of 18 % achieved after 1 year of the contract could be explained in part, by the removal of police officers and the employment of civilian staff at frequently less than half the cost (Plimmer and Warrell 2013).

It is as yet unknown as to whether these levels of cost savings can be sustained. Unison have for example highlighted the early savings achieved by contractors through the imposition of local market pay rates on civilian employees (Plimmer and Warrell 2013). Thus it becomes a matter of immediate interest to private contractors to move existing police staff from the police service to the company. In Cleveland under TUPE rules all staff were moved from the police authority to *Steria*. Any future civilian employees recruited through natural wastage would expect, however, to be paid at local market levels which would be substantially lower than current civilian staff rates (Loveday 2013).

Moreover after 10 years or less all civilian employees can expect to be paid at local market rates (Loveday 2013). In Lincolnshire G4S staff have taken over jobs formerly handled by police officers while around 575 civilian staff have been transferred from the police authority to G4S (Plimmer and Warrell 2013). While therefore the savings accruing to the police force are significant the costs of this process can be expected to fall very clearly on police staff, already the lowest paid sector within the police service (Loveday 2013).

Nor it would seem are errant private suppliers likely to be subject to any significant reprimand from a government clearly committed to the major expansion of private sector engagement with police support services. Thus *Serco* which earlier was involved in allegations of over-charging on prisoner escort contracts, has now been informed that it will be able to bid again in future for government contracts. G4S which has also been involved in alleged overcharging on electronic tagging and prisoner escort contracts is expected to be able to bid for new government contracts in the near future, subject of course, to the oversight of a crown representative (Travis 2014). It is also evident that the roll–out of outsourcing has much further to go. At least 10 other police forces are considering outsourcing arrangements where police custody centres and all IT programmes would be operated by private companies. By 2012 it was to be discovered that Thames Valley, West Mercia, Warwickshire, Staffordshire, Gloucestershire, Wiltshire and Hampshire police forces were engaged in tendering processes to outsource management of 30 custody suites and 600 cells. There is an expectation that over time private suppliers could be engaged in crime investigations, transporting suspects and managing intelligence (Telegraph

2012). Employing staff at significantly lower wage rates than those for either sworn officers or police staff will of course only serve to increase the potential profitability of contract arrangements for private suppliers. Yet the primary driver remains a continuing government commitment to a reduction in police expenditure where cuts to police central funding have been identified as standing at £ 2.1 billion for 2014–2015 compared to funding levels in 2010–2011 (HMIC 2014, p. 66).

As a result, outsourcing continues to be viewed by government and many members of ACPO (Association of Chief Police Officers) as the best alternative to reductions in police establishment and front-line provision of police services (Information Daily.com 2014). It is, of course, a position that is not entirely shared by the Police Federation which has condemned outsourcing as 'creeping privatisation'. Currently, however, the unfortunate excesses of a number of Federation members has led to both a highly critical independent review of its internal organisation (RSA 2014 Independent Review) and a potentially significant reduction in its influence over future police reform.

Moreover one balancing feature of the outsourcing process is the imposition of contractual accountability which remains an important feature of all outsourcing. Failure to comply with a contract or failure to fulfil contractual obligations can lead to substantial fines for the companies concerned. There is some evidence to suggest that contractual accountability can in fact lead to far greater responsiveness on the part of the supplier than might otherwise be achieved. As the recent heavy fines paid by both *Serco* and *G4S* demonstrate this may create more immediate contract compliance than formal, public accountability mechanisms. Interestingly some time ago courts in America were to explore the potential value of attacking the financial 'deep pocket 'of police departments where departments could be made subject to heavy financial penalties as a consequence of the professional failures of their officers (Loveday 1989).

Workforce Modernisation

Yet the current emphasis placed on outsourcing as the primary response to budget cuts has had, besides expanding the role of the private sector, a further impact. This relates to what appears to be the almost complete eclipse of the potential advantages and savings arising from the full implementation of the workforce modernisation programme tested very successfully at a number of demonstration sites prior to the arrival of the Coalition Government in 2010. Based upon the premise that much police work could be undertaken by non-sworn officers which could release serving police officers to deal with more complex cases it reflected a view best expressed in the HMIC Thematic report Modernising the Police service that fundamental change was necessary to improve the efficiency and effectiveness of the police service (HMIC Thematic 2004).

Mixed Economy Teams (METs)

Data coming from the demonstration sites proved to be overwhelmingly positive. The programme is based upon increased recruitment of civilian staff to whom are given a much wider range of policing responsibilities. Identified by way of 'mixed economy teams' (METs) consisting of constables and civilian investigative assistants, the innovative use of civilian staff in more numerous operational roles proved to be highly successful. In Surrey it was to be discovered that by increasing police support staff numbers it was found that a great deal more service delivery hours could be provided to Surrey residents (Loveday 2008a).

Moreover following analysis of crime resolution in the same county it was found that in only a small percentage of cases were the high level skills of specialists actually needed. This became particularly apparent in relation to the detective function. As a result many more investigative assistants were to be employed and made responsible for processing most volume crime in the force area. An initial evaluation of the METs suggested there had been big gains arising from their introduction and where the average investigation time had fallen from 26 to 15 days while the detection rate was to rise by 14 % (Loveday 2008a).

Very similar results were to arise in Bexley, another pilot site, where METs were to reduce the average investigation time per case from 50 to 16 days. A similar result was to be identified in relation to detections as a percentage of crime recorded. In the course of the METs experiment in Bexley, police staff made up a third of personnel employed in crime investigation teams. At this time further expansion was planned, based on the interesting fact that members of the public appeared to be quite happy to deal with any member of the MPS, whether police officers or police staff (Loveday 2008a).

Making volume crime a responsibility of METs in fact allowed professionally trained detectives to direct their attention to more serious offences. Further rationalisation of operational functions by way of greater division of labour was clearly identified as a significant contribution to increased efficiency and effectiveness within each police command (Loveday 2008a).

It remains a matter of speculation as to why the gains achieved at the Bexley site were to be thrown away as the METs experiment was subsequently closed down and all civilian investigators removed. It may have been a result of Police Federation pressure or the fact that this initiative had proved to be altogether too successful. Subject to debate in the House of Lords, no satisfactory explanation was ever to be provided for the decision of the MPS senior hierarchy to bring to an end the use of Investigative Support Officers and to close the site (House of Lords Hansard Debates, 20 March 2008, Col 380).

Despite the evident attempt to bury the good news within MPS it is clear that the demonstration sites have in fact proved to be highly instructive. They show that one clear way to improve future police effectiveness will be to significantly increase the number of civilian staff undertaking operational police roles. This of course raises the question of costs at a time of austerity. It is argued here that increasing police staff numbers would greatly enhance police visibility in the police area at a much lower cost. This could, moreover, be undertaken by a further reduction in police establishment which continues to be now, as in the past, a high cost and low value barrier to management flexibility.

Some evidence of this has been recently provided by the chief constable of Devon and Cornwall Police. He has recently argued that the extent of the cuts could leave his force 'operating only as a reactive force' working as an emergency service 'parked up in lay-bys ready to respond' (Sommers 2014a). This dire warning is based on the fact that cuts have lead to a reduction of police establishment from 3082 to 3047 sworn officers in a 6 month period ending September 2013. This does represent a fall of 422 police officers in the establishment figure of 3469 officers which pertained in 2011 (UK Police Directory 2011).

Yet no reference was to be made by the chief constable to any reduction in civilian staff numbers and the emphasis was placed solely on police officer establishment. This might be thought an unusual omission not least because civilian staff formerly constituted one third of the police force. This could be seen as, perhaps, more ironic in view of the need for greater flexibility demanded in response to current environment of austerity, where the effective deployment of resources becomes of paramount concern, not police establishment (Boyd et al. 2011). Elsewhere in Dyfed-Powys Police, the chief constable has decided to recruit 30 new police constables which he intends to pay for by reducing police staff numbers by 118 and making 55 police staff redundant while also encouraging voluntary redundancy applications (Sommers 2014b). This interesting decision may serve to highlight the limited horizons which continue to be exhibited within ACPO ranks.

Both cases do however serve to draw attention, yet again, to the very limited options currently open to police managers. In the absence of any power of compulsory severance being extended from police staff to police officers then retaining 'front line' policing can apparently only be achieved by eliminating staff that could offer high value and low cost, services. In its absence chief officers have to work within a very clearly defined straightjacket about which other than eliminating police staff, they can apparently do very little. This serves to also undermine any meaningful introduction of workforce modernisation which in an age of austerity has, it might be thought, an immediate application.

Police Force Collaboration

One further initiative with which some police forces appear to be struggling concerns collaborative arrangements between police forces. Recently HMIC have noted that some police forces were still finding it difficult to take full advantage of collaborative arrangements (Caswell 2014a). It is evident that collaboration provides a good way of making use of the advantages of the economies of scale. It also offers a meaningful and effective alternative to the costly process of police force amalgamation. While some forces are experiencing difficulties it is fair to say that others have been able to achieve considerable success in this area.

One example of this has proved to be the collaborative arrangements made between forces in the East Midlands where four police forces—Lincolnshire, Leicestershire, Northamptonshire and Nottinghamshire have been involved in a major collaborative project which while securing efficiencies 'will maintain the integrity of local policing' (Caswell 2014b). To date this has involved the development of close working relationships in relation to forensic services, command and control, public order, armed policing and strategic roads policing (Caswell 2014b).

It is fair to say that collaborative arrangements have been encouraged by the Centre for some time. In 2009 the Home Office and NPIA were to identify a range of possible collaborative links between forces involving a wide number of functions. In the North East for example Durham and Cleveland were to develop a joint firearms unit while in Wales the four forces were to develop collaborative approaches to the delivery of major crime serious and organised crime and cross border crime. In Surrey and Sussex a joint serious crime investigation team was to be established. A similar collaboration has been created between Essex and Kent police forces (Matrix Insight 2009).

Interestingly within the East Midland region where collaboration has been most advanced, the forces involved do not contemplate amalgamation. It is argued that the process can create strong alliances while also ensuring a continuing commitment to the local policing of each county (Caswell 2014b). The chief constable of Lincolnshire has recently argued in relation to regional collaboration that he believed that retaining the identity of forces was important and that in 5 years time he expected to see the same number of chief constables and PCCs as now. However he also noted that:

'What there cannot be is five different ways of doing functions that we can do together' (and that) 'we owe it to the public to make savings and to work together where this makes sense' (Caswell 2014b).

A New Dimension to Collaboration

The current move towards greater integration of strategic and other services between police forces is now well developed and a recent HMIC Report was to find that the pace and extent of collaboration was increasing (HMIC 2012, p. 8). However it is now also clear that the structure of collaboration and its extent can be expected to change quite dramatically in the future and go well beyond potential arrangements between police forces. Thus a number of PCCs have already identified the need for closer collaboration between all local emergency services where closer integration can achieve substantial savings (Policy Exchange 2013). Most recently the Policing Minister has highlighted the potential for collaboration 'in three dimensions' where future arrangements would include the police, wider blue light services and where the third dimension would be with other local partners such as councils (Address to the Association of PCCs 2014, Home Office).

The extension of collaborative arrangements to other public non emergency public agencies may have much to recommend it. One recent initiative undertaken by the Staffordshire PCC highlights the perceived need for this. A study undertaken in Staffordshire over an 8 week period drew attention to the amount of police time spent responding to issues of mental health in the community. It found that around 18 % of police time was taken up responding to incidents relating to mental health (Policy Exchange 2013, p. 33). The PCC was to note however that while police officers were often best placed to stabilise such incidents too often the specialist expertise and facilities needed to support individuals with complex conditions were not available and that 'individuals who had committed no offence could be potentially criminalised or their condition made significantly worse by being held in a custodial rather than a health orientated environment' (Policy Exchange 2013, p. 34). One result of this has been the decision to monitor the introduction of mental health workers at selected police stations and where collaboration would be encouraged between police health and social services (Policy Exchange 2013, p. 35).

It could be argued that a similar collaborative arrangement could be explored which involved police and local authorities in response to the overwhelming problem of anti-social behaviour (ASB) highlighted in HMICs 2010 Report (HMIC 2010). As the same report noted the response of the police was to identify ASB as a 'second order problem' and to relegate it as a low priority issue (HMIC 2010). This interesting police response to what very frequently constitutes a first order problem for both the public in general and victims in particular raises potentially interesting questions about future response to ASB and also resource allocation issues following on from that. Thus as with mental health so too with anti-social behaviour there is only a limited role for enforcement officers in responding to incidents (or not) rather than resolving the underlying problem. There may well therefore be a case for future reallocation of a level of resource away from law enforcement towards 'social support officers'. While the expanded use of PCSOs has of course better enabled the police to respond to local ASB problems it is evident that much more needs to be done (Blair 2009, p. 129).

This might be best achieved by a significant expansion of neighbourhood (or street) wardens employed by local authorities who could be expected to provide a long term presence in a problem area rather than the often reactive and limited response offered by the police. Moreover the presence of neighbourhood wardens might also be expected to ameliorate position of victims of ASB. Currently the use of law enforcement officers can often make a bad situation far worse, a consequence that police officers have themselves identified in seeking to deter victims from calling for police service. This may in part explain why in areas where demand for police service is highest police provision of service can be expected to be lowest and also the least effective (Loveday 1997, pp. 137–138).

Conclusion

Future police management in an age of austerity should be ready to experiment with innovative developments that provide a level of service expected of it by the public. As has been argued elsewhere, the debate cannot be about police establishment any longer but should concentrate on both police deployment and more effective resource allocation. If this approach is undertaken then police managers and PCCs will need to reassess future manpower configurations. If the evidence suggests that further reductions in police establishment when balanced by increases in non sworn civilian staff undertaking more operational roles could increase police effectiveness then this should be addressed. Nor is this a matter for future consideration as the value of work force modernisation has already been clearly identified.

Additionally in an environment that now increasingly recognises the significance and impact of antisocial behaviour on both individuals and communities there is a clear case for further evaluation of alternatives to a police response to it. The evidence suggests that the very identifiable limitations of a law enforcement approach needs to be finally acknowledged.

One solution could well be the substitution of high cost and low value law enforcement officers by high value but low cost neighbourhood wardens. These could provide the basis for both an effective collaboration between police and local authorities while also providing a more effective response to community demands and victims needs.

References

ACPO (2011). *UK police directory*. Brighton: Pavilion Publishing.
BBC West Midlands. (2012). PCC Bob Jones scraps business partnering plans. http://www.bbc.co.uk/news/uk-england-birmingham-20442968.
Blair, I. (2009). *Policing controversy*. London: Profile Books.
Boyd, E., Geoghegan, R., & Gibbs, B. (2011). *Cost of the cops: Manpower and deployment in policing*. London: Policy Exchange.
Caswell, J. (2014). Major blow to G4S as police multimillion-pound deal to outsource services collapses. *The Independent*, 30th November 2013.
Caswell, C. (2014a). Regional collaboration 'a model for the future'. *Police Oracle*. 13th February.
Caswell, C. (2014b). HMIC: Forces still struggling with collaboration. *Police Oracle*. 13th March.
Ford, R. (2013). We fiddled our crime numbers, admit police. *The Times*. 20th November 2013.
HMIC Thematic. (2004). *Modernising the police service*. London: Home Office.
HMIC. (2010). Stop the Rot. Anti-Social Behaviour in England and Wales, Home Office, London.
HMIC. (2012). *Policing in austerity: One year on, HMIC*. London: Home Office.
HMIC. (2014). *State of policing*. London: Annual Assessment of Policing in England and Wales, HMIC.
Home Office. (2014). *Police Grant (England and Wales)*. London: The Police Grant Report 2014/15, HC 1043, Stationary Office.
House of Lords. (2008). *Hansard Debates*. 20th March 2008. Col 380.
Lincolnshire Police Authority. (2011). Outsourcing decision. http:/http:lincs.police.uk/News-Centre/news-Releases/21-12-2001 Police Authority-outs. Accessed 14 Oct 2015.

Loveday, B. (1989). Recent developments in police complaints procedure: Britain and North America. *Local Government Studies, 15* (3), 25–57.

Loveday, B. (1997). Crime, policing and the provision of service. In P. Francis, P. Davies, & V. Jupp (Eds.), *Policing futures, the police law enforcement and the 21st Century.* Basingstoke Hants: Macmillan.

Loveday, B. (2006). Policing performance. *International Journal of Police Science and Management, 8*(3), 282–292.

Loveday, B. (2008a). Workforce modernisation in the police service. *International Journal of Police Science and Management, 10*(2), 136–144.

Loveday, B. (2008b). Workforce modernisation and future resilience within the Police Service in England and Wales. *The Police Journal, 81*(1), 62–81.

Loveday, B. (2013). Police reform in England and Wales: A new dimension in accountability and service delivery in the 21st century. In N. Fyfe, J. Terpstra, & P. Tops (Eds.), *Centralising forces.* The Hague: Eleven International Publishing.

Martis, R. (2014). Compulsory severance: Fed reps voice caution. *Police Oracle.* 17th February 2014.

Matrix Insight. (2009). *Protective services demonstration sites evaluation.* London: Matrix Consultancy.

Muir, H. (2014). Diary. *The Guardian.* 11th March 2014.

Plimmer, G., & Warrell, H. (2013). Police Hail resumption of outsourcing contract. *Financial Times.* 24th June 2013.

Policy Exchange. (2011). Cost of the cops. Manpower and deployment in policing, Policy Exchange London.

Policing Minister. (2014). *Address to Association of PCCs.* London: Home Office.

Policy Exchange. (2013). *The Pioneers, PCCs one year on, A collection of essays.* London: Policy Exchange.

RSA (2014). *Police federation Independent review Final report The trusted voice for frontline officers.* London: RSA.

Sommers, J. (2014a). Chief: My force struggling under budget cuts. *Police Oracle.* 18th March 2014.

Sommers, J. (2014b). Force confirms restructure redundancies. *Police Oracle.* 8th January 2014.

The Information.Daily.com. (2014). Police Advised how to outsource services as cuts bite. http:/www.theinformationdaily.com/2013/07/08/police-advised-how-to-outsource-ser. Accessed 10 April 2015.

The Telegraph. (2012). Police privatisation to spread says G4S executive. *Telegraph Reporters.* 21st June 2012.

Travis, A. (2014). G4S still at risk of criminal proceedings. *The Guardian,* 12th March 2014.

Winsor Report. (2012). *Independent review of police officer and staff remuneration and conditions, Final Report Cm 8325-1.* Stationary Office: London.

Barry Loveday is a Reader in Criminal Justice at Portsmouth University since 1994. He was Principal Lecturer in Criminal Justice at Birmingham City University from 1979–1994. He has been involved with research into police effectiveness and police management over many years and has been an adviser to the Local Government Associations' Community Safety Panel; He has contributed to the work on policing for both the IPPR and Policy Exchange Think Tanks and latterly was an adviser to the PMs Strategy Unit under New Labour. He has published extensively on policing and in particular the impact of performance management, civilianisation, workforce modernisation and reform of police governance in England and Wales. He is currently engaged in evaluating the potential expansion of the role of neighbourhood wardens in response to the continuing challenge of anti –social behaviour in areas experiencing high levels of deprivation as an alternative to police service intervention.

Chapter 11
Personal Resilience and Policing

Jonathan Smith and Ginger Charles

Introduction

Major changes in the police landscape internationally have been seen in recent years. Huge cuts in funding; significant reductions in both police officers and staff; looking to do more with less; changes in governance; mergers between forces, sometimes even into one large national police service; increases in the pace and amount of change; and shifts in the nature of crime and ways of tackling this are just some examples globally (Crime and Policing Group 2011; Wiharta et al. 2012; National Audit office 2014).

What can often be forgotten though in this process of change are those within these police organisations—leaders, police officers and staff at every level. We are concerned about how they are managing to cope with all this change and uncertainty. More so, how are they doing anything more than just hunkering down as a reaction to these changes and just focusing on survival? How do those working in the police thrive, grow and prosper within this environment of constant challenge and change? Large questions and not just moral ones related to individuals' health and well-being, but also of major organisational significance in terms of performance, employee engagement, costs of ill health and potential litigation claims.

J. Smith (✉)
Devon and Cornwall Police, Middlemoor, Exeter, Devon. EX27HQ, UK
e-mail: jonathan.smith3@devonandcornwall.pnn.police.uk

G. Charles
Institute for Spirituality and Policing, Modesto, California, USA
e-mail: gingercharles@me.com

G. Charles
Modesto Junior College, Modesto, California, USA
e-mail: gingercharles@me.com

© Springer International Publishing Switzerland 2015
P. Wankhade, D. Weir (eds.), *Police Services*, DOI 10.1007/978-3-319-16568-4_11

In this chapter we seek to explore some of the issues involved here through the lens of resilience. We will draw on our own research and experiences of working within the police in both the UK and USA for a combined period of over 40 years. We've been conducting research since 2000 with well over a 150 police officers related to resilience, well-being, and how officers and police leaders cope with the demanding nature of their job. This is summarised in Smith and Charles (2010; 2013). We will begin this chapter by defining resilience, outline why this may be an important focus, and explore stress and how stress and resilience are connected. We then go on to detail some of the research in this area. From this an emphasis on holistic resilience emerges. We will outline what this is and the key components to it. Then we will outline some key points concerning how holistic resilience may prove useful and how it may be further developed within the police organisation as a way of enabling all who work there to thrive and grow in the constantly changing and challenging environment.

What is Resilience?

According to Haglund et al. (2007, p. 899) resilience refers to the 'ability to successfully adapt to stressors, maintaining psychological well-being in the face of adversity'. Successfully adapting to a variety of stressors certainly seems to be an important skill that is needed for those in policing, particularly in the context of the discussion in the previous section. Though we argue in our work that the vast majority of police officers and staff are capable of handling adversity and stressors, our focus is on how resilient officers do this and what others can learn from this.

Luthans (2002, p. 702) also refers to the psychological aspects to resilience when he talks of resilience as the 'positive psychological capacity to rebound or bounce back from adversity, uncertainty, conflict, failure or even positive change, progress and increased responsibility'. Luthans' definition extends our thinking about resilience to not just being required in the face of adversity, but to its need in both positive and negative experiences at work. Luthans also highlights the important 'bouncing back' aspect of resilience, which emphasises that resilient individuals and organisations are not necessarily those that never fail or wander from the right direction. It gives us hope in that we do not have to be superhuman and recognises that we are all human and that on some occasions we can falter, will struggle, or feel overwhelmed and can wander from the right path. Luthans shows that resilience is more about the ability to get up again after a setback and carry on. This faltering could be over a short-term issue, or over a longer-term period. This 'bouncing-back' aspect of resilience has certainly been seen many times in our own research. The most recent study involves 11 police officers from various agencies in Colorado in the United States (Charles et al. 2014). The first author of this study has followed these officers through the last few years of their career. We found that almost every one of them has struggled or faltered at some point with a significant issue such as addiction, divorce, death of a loved one, or reassignment in their career. All the participants though have found ways of overcoming the obstacles they experienced and of regaining their footing on the path. Interestingly the recognition of faltering often involved the officers being reprimanded for their behaviour by their supervisor in their work setting. The officers and immediate supervisors would then work together to correct the behaviour and help the officer. The organisation thus helped these officers recognise and correct their destructive behaviour. Humility and insight were paramount to these law enforcement officers' resiliency.

Research by Brigadier General Cornum (2012), who until recently led the $ 125 million emotional fitness regime for the US military, suggests that the things that enable a person to '*bounce back*' are not all due to an individual's make-up: effective coping strategies can be learned and developed. Everyone has the ability to develop resilience.

A lot of the research on personal resilience has focused on the emergency and caring services, probably because more demand for effective coping strategies are evident here with the high levels of stress experienced. McAllister and McKinnon (2008, p. 2) for example argue that 'learning about and applying strategies of resilience are vital and should be a key component of all health curricula for health professionals'. Examples of this type of research can be seen in the police, army, ambulance service, nursing, and social work.

The definitions from Haglund et al. (2007) and Luthans (2002) highlight the psychological aspects to resilience. Much of the work on personal resilience also focuses on emotional resilience (Paton 2006; Gilmartin 2002). Emotional resilience links people's physical and emotional reactions, seeks to explain why the body reacts in the way it does and offers useful strategies to help overcome the negative reactions and effects. Emotions are undoubtedly a very important element to resilience, but they do not cover the complete picture. Beddoes-Jones (2012, p. 46) extends this analysis and highlights the physical, mental and emotional aspects to resilience, introducing more of a holistic perspective. Richardson (2002) and Cornum (2012) are some of the few to take the holistic exploration still further and include the spiritual dimension as an important aspect to resilience.

The Need for Resilience

Resilience is receiving a great deal of attention currently, both within the police and more broadly, but it is still an underexplored topic particularly within the work and policing contexts. There is still much to be done, much to understand. It is an important and necessary focus for managers and HR professionals however, chiefly because of the large number of changes and levels of uncertainty of the type we outlined at the start of this chapter. This is resulting in significant amounts of stress being experienced within the workplace, which is having some major negative impacts. Stress is the 'Health Epidemic of the twenty-first Century' according to the World Health Organisation (2013), and is estimated to be costing American businesses alone $ 300 billion a year. It is a major threat to the health and well-being of people at work across the world. Every year, according to Black and Frost (2011), 140 million days are lost to sickness in the UK, with employers paying £ 9 billion and the State £ 13 billion per year on health-related benefits. For each year over the last 5 years, work-related stress, depression or anxiety has been the single most reported complaint (Health and Safety Executive (HSE) 2008).

We argue that if a greater understanding of resilience and the relationship between resilience and stress can be achieved, then managers and HR professionals will be better able to proactively implement support and training interventions to assist employees to cope more effectively with the stress that is inherent in today's workplaces, including police workplaces. In addition to interventions that assist individuals to build their resilience we argue that organisations can embed policies, practices and a culture to enable the organisation as a whole to be more resilient in coping with the various stressors employees encounter.

Holistic Resilience

As we have said, much of the work so far has focused on various single aspects of resilience including emotional and psychological. We see a broader range of issues now emerging which are connected to resilience. We thus argue for a more holistic view of resilience, as identified by Richardson (2002, p. 310). Although more work is required as to all the specific aspects that are covered by this holistic resilience, we use the Global Fitness Framework (GFF) shown in Fig. 11.1, to illustrate some of the key points.

The GFF is a holistic framework developed by Rayment and Smith (2013). This framework highlights three areas to a holistic perspective—Organic Level, Fitness Plane and Holistic Depth, and three elements in each of these. At the Organic Level it highlights that the focus can be at the individual level, the group (which can be anything from a small team to the organisation) and the societal level. The Fitness

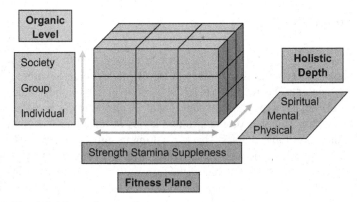

Fig. 11.1 The global fitness framework

Plane focuses on fitness, and fitness for purpose, which provides both a flexible and dynamic orientation and terms which may be more familiar within the policing context. There are many similarities between fitness and resilience, particularly related to the elements of strength, stamina and suppleness identified in Fig. 11.1. The Holistic Depth element of the GFF identifies physical, mental and spiritual aspects. Rayment and Smith (2013) also consider emotional aspects and argue that emotions are actually formed of the physical, mental and spiritual components that are explicitly identified within the GFF. We recognise that drawing distinctions, as is done in the GFF, between mind, body and spirit, is a simplification of reality, and can give the impression that spirituality is simply just one discrete element of a whole. It is more complex than this, but it is a convenient, simple and clear way to highlight the different aspects in a holistic approach.

The physical aspects to resilience at the individual level have perhaps received the most attention to date and include the physical signs and symptoms of stress and, in terms of coping strategies, such things as the importance or exercise, healthy eating and sufficient rest and sleep. The mental components at the individual level include knowledge and understanding of the signs and symptoms of stress, the positive aspects to stress, the health dangers of too much stress, and again ways of building resilience including positive thinking and developing a positive mental attitude. It is the spiritual aspects however which we are identifying as the most under-explored and contentious aspects of resilience, and yet one of the most significant and exciting (see Smith and Charles 2013). We explore this further within a policing context in the next section.

The GFF also identifies there are physical, mental and spiritual aspects to resilience at both the organisational and societal levels, and it is in these areas that most work is still to be done. We argue though that police leaders can build and embed policies, practices and a culture that enables the organisation as a whole to be more resilient.

The Spiritual Aspects of Resilience

According to Smith (2009) there is a growing awareness of the importance and significance of the spiritual dimension within policing. In the UK, Her Majesty's Inspectorate of Constabulary (HMIC) recognised the importance of this issue back in 2003. There is a section in its 2003 report (HMIC 2003, p. 119) which specifically relates to the spiritual needs of staff in the police service. This stated:

> In the context of dealing with the stresses and strains of diversity, attention needs to be given to the spiritual needs of people.

HMIC (2003, p. 120) also made a clear recommendation on this issue:

> HM Inspector recommends that all forces have resources in place to meet the spiritual needs of police officers and police staff, while respecting the diversity of faiths and beliefs both inside the service and in the communities which they serve.

More recently the Equality Act (2010) places a duty on public authorities to promote better understanding between people who hold different faiths, and those who hold none. Perhaps more importantly though, if the fundamental challenges of policing are considered—dealing with death, right v wrong, being ostracised by communities, building relationships and embracing diversity—many are fundamentally spiritual challenges. As a result it would seem logical and worthy of further consideration as to whether the most effective ways of coping with these fundamental spiritual challenges could include consideration of the spiritual.

The spiritual dimension is a complex, and controversial area though (non more so than within the police), and is often overlooked within holistic approaches, although it is increasingly being identified as a vital element which can have a large influence on the physical, mental and emotional aspects of work (see for example Rayment and Smith 2013, p. 12). Unfortunately the majority of studies (for example Richardson (2002) and Cornum (2012) that explore spirituality and resilience treat spirituality as a single entity which is easily measured and controlled. Spirituality is in reality a complex, multi-dimensional phenomenon. Hence research which embraces a broad interpretation of spirituality is important in order to expand our understanding. There are some (such as Conger et al. 1994; Lantos 1999) who interpret spirituality using just a religious definition. This narrow religious interpretation of spirituality, often seen in America and the UK as a Christian interpretation, is not appropriate for the police services that pride themselves on their anti-discriminatory practices. Of course a religious interpretation is an important perspective because many people do see spirituality and religion as the same thing, and so different religious interpretations do need to be included as part of a much broader interpretation of spirituality.

Spirituality is not something that can easily be defined. People's understanding of spirituality is more likely to unfold over time through discussion, and from finding its meaning in practice. As a result there are likely to be many different perspectives of spirituality that emerge. There is also a danger in the work context of simply trying to use it as a tool for gaining greater engagement, commitment, or productivity. Approaching spirituality in this way may make it easier to measure, specify, and sell, but employees are likely to very quickly see through this motive and it is unlikely to work for long.

Meaning

In many explorations of spirituality (see examples in Robinson and Smith 2014), the issue of meaning is prominent. This relates to people striving for some purpose and meaning to their lives. There is no single meaning in life, and the search of meaning is a personal one. However the meaning and purpose discussed here is not purely for personal or material gain, it refers more to work that contributes to something bigger than the individual—serving others, making a difference, contributing to a greater good or higher goal. This meaning is linked to a sense of worth and of feeling valued. Within a work context, meaning is also linked to creating a purpose for the organisation, helping people make sense of their lives and showing how their work contributes to the organisation's and their own purpose in life.

Individual's views of meaning are very much linked to and develop from a person's sense of calling to undertake a particular task or role, which Conklin (2013) explores, and which we see a great deal of within the police (Smith and Charles 2010, p. 325). Conklin (2013, p. 300) highlights the importance of meaning for motivation and in coping with stress. The issue of meaning is also identified by the Chartered Institute of Personnel & Development (CIPD) (2011) as being important to employees in developing quality employment relationships.

Given the challenges and situations regularly being dealt with by the police, questions of meaning are often raised and seem particularly significant in this context. As a result discussions to align individual, organisational and the different stakeholder perspectives of meaning are in some ways perhaps easier within the police.

Connection

Another fundamental aspect related to spirituality that comes out of the literature is the concept of connectedness (see examples in Robinson and Smith 2014). Smith (2005) identifies a number of possible vertical and horizontal connections here including 'themselves, other people, nature, the universe, a god, or some other supernatural power'. Connecting with other people is a key motivator for many in actually going to work, and seems particularly relevant for the policing role. Robinson and Smith (2014) point out that the different connections noted above by Smith (2005) are not just simply and harmoniously integrated purely through a focuses on spirituality. On the contrary, they point out; spirituality is a continuing, and often messy, dialogue between these aspects.

Within policing this valuing of other perspectives is key and the cornerstone of both embracing diversity and of policing by consent. It can also be where many organisational initiatives fall down, in that they are only focused on the organisation and its members. The many other different stakeholders that are involved—including community, nature, the environment, and planet—can be overlooked. Relationships with, and valuing of communities, faiths and beliefs, both locally, national and international are though key to both policing, policing by consent and embracing of diversity, as the HMIC (2003, p. 120) and Equality Act (2010) highlight. Exploring relationships with others outside of the police organisation and questioning the ultimate meaning and purpose of the police service would also seem to help facilitate the partnership working with other public sector agencies such as Fire and Rescue Services, probation, the voluntary sector, county community safety officers, the Home Office, health services staff and the prison service that are seeing increasing emphasis (Meaklim and Sims 2011).

Isolation

Another particularly significant issue for the police in relation to the connectedness aspect to spirituality and resilience is isolation. Police officers are sworn and trained to protect and serve the citizens of the community, yet those citizens may also be the enemy. In their research Smith and Charles (2010, p. 328) found that as a result of this dynamic officers can become overly suspicious of others and find it difficult to disclose their feelings. For their own safety officers can isolate themselves from people outside the law enforcement community, and this can become more pronounced the longer an officer serves. According to Violanti and Paton (1999), the law enforcement community encourages solidarity among its officers as a way of protecting the group from those outside the profession who are perceived as unable to understand. Nickels and Verma (2008, p. 204) also found this solidarity and collegiality common across the police officers they studied in Canada, India and Japan. Smith's and Charles' (2010, p. 329) finding is that the police can have powerful clannish tendencies and beliefs. Some of these beliefs are intrinsic in the law enforcement community because of the dependence upon each other to survive critical incidents, attack and life and death conflicts. As a result, officers can begin to associate only with other officers (socialising, drinking, and working out in gyms with other officers) and may even reside in police officer-dominated neighbourhoods, gradually losing contact with others outside the profession, until the only relationships available to them are those with other police officers. According to Smith and Charles (2010, p. 329) this primary coping resource constricts cognitive flexibility and can remove officers from other valuable social roles that may provide helpful coping mechanisms. Due to this internal pressure, an unwillingness to seek help from the many support facilities available within the police services can develop.

The police environment is often identified as a male dominated world, emphasising a 'culture of toughness', based on physical strength and aggression (Carlier 1999; Violanti 1999). Like military combat, police work involves a continual sense of danger from an unknown enemy, constantly witnessing violence and death, experiencing a depersonalisation of emotion and the belief in a lack of public support. Police officers can therefore experience pressures to isolate themselves from people outside the organisation as well as isolate themselves from their feelings and emotions. This all highlights that the connectedness, and linked isolation element, of spirituality may be an important aspect of building resilience within a policing environment.

In summary, this exploration of spirituality highlights its complex, contentious and multi-dimensional nature. Some prefer to avoid these conflicts and tensions and leave considerations of a spiritual nature outside of the work environment. We have seen though that within a work and policing context there are many aspects to spirituality that appear to be of relevance in this exploration of resilience. Four key aspects have been highlighted in this exploration as being important in a view of spirituality related to resilience that is appropriate for the contemporary police workplace. Firstly explorations of spirituality need to be inclusive. Spirituality is a broad, multidimensional concept and in today's multi-cultural, diverse police work-places it is important to embrace a multitude of different interpretations, including institutionalised religions as particular but not all expressions of spirituality. Secondly an important aspect of spirituality in connection to resilience is in helping to find meaning. This is linked to a person's sense of calling to undertake a particular task or role, and to a sense of worth. Thirdly the importance of connectedness, which seems particularly significant for the police, and can be a key motivator for many in going to work. Finally spirituality needs to be viewed as part of a holistic perspective. We argue there are physical, mental emotional as well as spiritual components to resilience, and all these are important and need to be considered as well as their interaction and the whole.

Benefits of Resilience

Having discussed the appreciation of resilience and the different aspects that make it up, we turn our attention to the possible benefits of resilience in the policing context. We identified something of this in the exploration earlier in this chapter regarding stress. If building greater resilience can help to militate even a small part of this stress and reduce the individual and organisational costs involved, it can result in significant savings. To illustrate the savings, we draw on an on-going study into stress, burnout and Post Traumatic Stress Disorder (PTSD) by Liddell (2013). This is the largest survey of police forces in England in this area that has so far been conducted, and involves some 350 responses from various members of police forces. Liddell's findings include:

- 60 % of respondents say they feel like they have no one to talk to;
- 40 % of respondents are deemed to be at medium or high risk of Burnout;
- 42 % of respondents have been signed off work with stress one or more times;
- 13 % of respondents have been signed off work with PTSD one or more times, usually for 4+ months costing over £ 11k per officer per instance, and;
- 79 % of officers feel that their Force does not do enough to support them after traumatic incidents.

Liddell estimates the cost of this to police forces in England alone to be just under £ 100 million per year. Although there are some methodological weaknesses with the research, primarily in the sample selection, the results show significant individual and organisational costs, including financial ones from the effects of police work.

There is a growing body of evidence suggesting that there are a range of benefits that can be realised from greater levels of personal resilience. Mallack (1998) and Zander and Hutton (2010) argue that strong personal resilience can militate against the effects of stress. There are benefits for people who work in the police, police leaders, police services, communities and wider society. These benefits relate to enabling people to cope better with the stresses they encounter both within their police work, and also life outside of work. Reduced levels of stress, burnout and incidents of PTSD, illness resulting from stress and exposure to traumatic events, reduced time off sick, increased levels of well-being, engagement and productivity are all factors which can result from increased levels of resilience and which impact significantly on individuals, the police service, and the levels of service provided to the public. Given the current austere environment in which many police organisations are operating within, these benefits are of real significance.

A range of benefits have also been identified which relate specifically to the impact of spirituality on health and well-being at work. From a systematic review of studies between 1806–2009, Koenig (2011) claims religious involvement is related to greater well-being and happiness, lesser depression & faster recovery from depression, lesser suicide rates and more negative attitudes toward suicide, and significantly more forgiveness. Koenig does link these findings to religious involvement but uses the terms spirituality and religion interchangeably. Care has to be taken with the research evidence that is presented in this area however as there are a number of weaknesses with some of the research, particularly connected to how spirituality is viewed and measured as we have discussed previously. There also tends to be a large focus on benefits, without many difficulties or problems being identified. The reader is directed to Robinson and Smith (2014) for a fuller critical analysis of the research, and an overview of the benefits and difficulties that have been identified.

What can be Done to Develop Resilience in the Police Environment?

Fortunately there is something that both individuals and organisations can do here as it seems people can be taught and encouraged to become more resilient. The first point, as we emphasised earlier in the chapter, is that we believe the majority of police officers and staff are very resilient and are able to cope effectively with the adversity and stressors they regularly encounter (see Smith and Charles 2010). If this is the case, the approach for developing resilience further must involve learning from these resilient officers across the world and disseminating the strategies that have been found to be successful specifically within the policing environment.

What is known about resilience and coping, and its relationships to stress and trauma provides a number of suggestions for strategies and solutions. One important aspect here seems to be about developing proactive strategies, rather than leaving it until people experience problems, when it can take much longer, and be more difficult and costly to resolve. Zander's and Hutton's (2010, p. 99) research in the related nursing profession, identifies a diversity of strategies used by nurses to enable them to cope with the stresses they encounter, and as a result the need for the organisation to offer a variety of strategies for them to choose from. Some of the most common strategies that emerge from Zander's and Hutton's (2010) research are spirituality and religion, social support, emotional expression, reflection, and problem solving. Generally from our analysis there seems to be a range of things that can be done to enhance personal resilience. These might be linked to the GFF in Fig. 11.1. Firstly, at the individual level, physical features might include regular physical exercise, diet and good sleep. Having a lack of these three important aspects can undermine physical health and it can also impact on other levels in the GFF, such as poor or illogical decision-making, and weaker mental and emotional wellbeing for instance. At the cognitive level, self-awareness and reflection are two of the keys—knowing and recognising the signs and symptoms of stress, and its sources, knowing what can be done about these, and taking action early to address them. At the spiritual level, providing opportunities and encouragement for people to reflect on the bigger questions in life—like the meaning of their life and how the work they are doing links to this—can be helpful. Working to develop good social support structure, both within and outside the police community also appear beneficial.

At the team and organisational level in the GFF, particularly related to the police service, our analysis reveals much can be done. The physical level of finance includes recognising the benefits and cost saving of investing in workplace health and employee wellbeing. Investing in offering health food in our canteens, time to eat and drink, gyms, opportunities and facilities to undertake physical exercise. Much of the work at the cognitive level is about creating an environment and culture where is it acceptable to discuss resilience and the challenges connected to this. An environment that offers access to specialist physical, psychological and spiritual support can help people feel able to access the extensive support that is very often provided by forces such as Counselling, TRiM (Trauma Risk incident Management) and critical incident debriefing, and which encourages early intervention to reduce risk factors and build a resilient workforce. The line manager also plays a vital role in helping to build resilience in the organisation. By knowing and looking out for early signs of distress or changes in behaviour or performance, a good manager can prevent absenteeism, ill-health, and loss of talent. At the spiritual level an organisation can engage employees more in discussions about vision and values, and work towards aligning individual's and the organisation's sense of larger purpose and value.

The different approaches highlighted here, all argue the need for support and training. This training is at every level within police forces and for all who work here; from new recruits to the most senior leaders; for police officers, staff, leaders, volunteers; and also their families. Training needs to include discussions on the challenges of policing and its possible impact on individuals, as well as exploring the importance of resilience and how the various aspects of holistic resilience can be developed.

Conclusion

It is clear that there are many challenges facing police services around the world. These challenges are impacting directly, and not always positively, on the people who work within these organisations. Increasing levels of stress and burnout are being seen. In this chapter we have explored how resilience may be useful in assisting people to not only cope with these challenges but thrive and prosper in this environment of uncertainty and rapid and constant challenge and change.

We have developed further the idea of holistic resilience, and explored the component parts to this, using a holistic framework called the Global Fitness Framework to assist. We have then explored some of the benefits to developing greater resilience at the level of the individual, organisation and at the societal level. We have concluded our discussion with an exploration of how the different elements to resilience might be developed by police organisations.

There is still much research needed though to understand resilience more fully in respect to the policing context. Research for instance which explores how both individuals and police organisations can further develop their resilience, and which articulates the benefits for both individuals, the police service and community it serves from doing this.

Given the limited attention currently devoted to resilience, research, training and discussion of these issues with the police it seems there may be substantial benefits to be gained from a greater focus on resilience in the police. These benefits are likely to include reduced costs for forces attributed to stress, burnout and attrition of police officers and staff. More importantly though support and training connected to resilience may assist to better prepare and protect the well-being of these ordinary people who have volunteered for the extraordinary vocation of service and protection.

Implications for Policing and Practice

This exploration raises significant implications for the police services. People working in these organisations are experiencing high levels of stress, which can impact on levels of ill health and sickness, burnout and incidents of PTSD. There are huge costs for individuals and organisations from this, which are much more than just financial costs. They also leave organisations increasingly vulnerable from litigation claims against them for not doing more to protect the psychological safety of the people who work there. There are larger moral questions too and nobody wants organisations that harms the people who work there when more could have been done to protect them. Great efforts are being placed on physically protecting officers but we believe more can be done proactively to provide greater psychological safety to police officers and staff. As well as the moral questions this answers it will also lead to high performing organisations and greater levels of service and satisfaction for the public. Now that is something that is meaningful to us all!

References

Beddoes-Jones, F. (2012). Authentic leadership: The key to building trust. *People Management*, August, 44–47.

Black, C., & Frost, D. (2011). *Health at work- an independent review of sickness absence*. Norwich: TSO.

Carlier, I. V. E. (1999). Finding meaning in police traumas. In J. M. Violanti & D. Paton (Eds.), *Police trauma: Psychological aftermath of civilian combat* (pp. 227–233). Springfield: Charles C. Thomas.

Charles, G. L., Travis, F., & Smith, J. A. (2014). Policing and spirituality: Their impact on brain integration and consciousness. *Journal of Management, Spirituality and Religion, 11*(3), 230–244.

CIPD. (2011). *Sustainable organisational performance. What really makes the difference?* London: Chartered Institute of Personnel Development.

Conger, J. A., et al. (1994). *Spirit at work: Discovering the spirituality in leadership*. San Francisco: Jossey-Bass.

Conklin, T. A. (2013). Work worth doing: A phenomenological study of the experience of discovering and following one's calling. *Journal of Management Inquiry, 21*(3), 298–317.

Cornum, R. (7 February 2012). Can we teach resilience? Brigadier General Rhonda Cornum on emotional fitness. Presentation at the young foundation, London. http://www.youngfoundation.org/general-/-all/events/can-we-teach-resilience-brigadier-general-rhonda-cornum-emotional-fitness. Accessed 25 Oct 2012.

Crime and Policing Group. (2011). https://www.gov.uk/government/uploads/. Accessed 31 Aug 2014.

Equality Act. (2010). http://www.legislation.gov.uk/ukpga/2010/15/contents. Accessed 19 Feb 2014.

Gilmartin, K. M. (2002). *Emotional survival for law enforcement: A guide for officers and their families*. Tuscon: E-S Press.

Haglund, M. E., Nestadt, P. S., Cooper, N. S., Southwick, S. M., & Charney, D. S. (2007). Psychobiological mechanisms of resilience: Relevance to prevention and treatment of stress-related psychopathology. *Development and Psychopathology, 19*(3), 889–920.

Health and Safety Executive (HSE). (2008). *Health and safety statistics 2008/9*. Suffolk: HSE.

Her Majesty's Inspectorate of Constabulary (HMIC). (2003). *Diversity matters*, Home Office Communication Directorate.

Koenig, H. (2011). *Handbook of religion and health* (2nd ed.). Oxford: Oxford University Press.

Lantos, G. P. (1999). Motivating moral corporate behavior. *Journal of Consumer Marketing, 16*(3), 395–407.

Liddell, E. (2013). *Prevalence on PTSD, compassion fatigue and burnout in the emergency services*. Presentation to the police federation health and safety conference 30th September. Police Federation Headquarters Leatherhead.

Luthans, F. (2002). The need for and meaning of positive organizational behavior. *Journal of Organizational Behaviour, 23*, 695–706.

Mallack, L. (1998). Putting organisational resilience to work. *Industrial Management, 40*(6), 8–14.

McAllister, M., & McKinnon, J. (2008). The importance of teaching and learning resilience in the health disciplines: A critical review of the literature. *Nurse Education Today, 29*(4), 371–379.

Meaklim, T., & Sims, J. (2011). Leading powerful partnerships- a new model of public sector leadership development. *International Journal of Leadership in Public Services, 7*(1), 22–31.

National Audit Office. (2014). The criminal justice system: Landscape review http://www.nao.org.uk/report/the-criminal-justice-system-landscape-review/ Accessed 31 Aug 2014

Nickels, E., & Verma, A. (2008). Dimensions of police culture: A study in Canada, India and Japan. *Policng: An International Journal of Police Strategies & Management, 31*(2), 186–209.

Paton, D. (2006). Critical incident stress risk in police officers: Managing resilience and vulnerability. *Traumatology, 12* (3), 198–206.

Rayment, J. J., & Smith, J. A. (2013). A holistic framework for leaders in a wicked world. *Journal of Finance and Management in Public Services, 11*(2), 1–19.

Richardson, G. E. (2002). The metatheory of resilience and resiliency. *Journal of Clinical Psychology, 58*(3), 307–321.

Robinson, S., & Smith, J. A. (2014). *Co-charismatic leadership: Critical perspectives on spirituality, ethics and leadership*. Oxford: Peter Lang.

Smith, J. A. (2005). *Training for the whole person: An exploration of possibilities for enhancing the spiritual dimension of police training*. PhD dissertation, University of Hull, Hull.

Smith, J. A. (2009). Police training for the whole person. *FBI Law Enforcement Bulletin, 78*(11), 1–8.

Smith, J. A., & Charles, G. (2010). The relevance of spirituality in policing: A dual analysis. *International Journal of Police Science and Management, 12*(3), 320–338.

Smith, J. A., & Charles, G. (2013). *Developing leadership resilience: Lessons from the policing frontline*. Farnham: Ashgate Publishing Ltd.

Violanti, J. M. (1999). Trauma in police work: A psychosocial model. In J. M. Violanti & D. Paton (Eds.), *Police trauma: Psychological aftermath of civilian combat*. Springfield: Charles C. Thomas.

Violanti, J., & Paton, D. (1999). *Police trauma: Psychological aftermath of civilian combat*. Springfield: Charles C. Thomas.

Wiharta, S., Melvin, N., & Avezov, X. (2012). The new geopolitics of peace operations. Mapping the emerging landscape. Stockholm International Peace Research Institute. www.sipri.org/research/conflict/pko/other. Accessed 31 Aug 2014

World Health Organisation (WHO). (2013). http://www.who.int/publications/en/. Accessed 19 Feb 2014

Zander, M., Hutton, A., & King, L. (2010). Coping and resilience factors in pediatric oncology nurses CE. *Journal of Pediatric Oncology Nursing, 27*(2), 94–108.

Dr. Jonathan Smith Chartered FCIPD is the Leadership Development Manager at Devon and Cornwall Police. Prior to this he was a Senior Lecturer at the Lord Ashcroft International Business School at Anglia Ruskin University, and prior to this a Director of Studies at the NPIA. He is a Fellow of the Leadership Trust, Member of the International Academic Advisory Board on Leadership in FE, Associate of the Centre for Governance, Leadership and Global Responsibility at Leeds Beckett University, Director of the Institute for Spirituality in Policing, and Member of the CIPD's Membership and Professional Development Committee. Co-author of many journal articles and books on leadership and policing including MisLeadership (2010), Ethics in Human Resource Management (2013), Developing Leadership Resilience: Lessons from the Policing Frontline (2013) and his latest book Co-Charismatic Leadership: Critical Perspectives on Spirituality, Ethics and Leadership (2014).

Prof. Dr. Ginger Charles has worked as a police officer in the United States since 1986. As a police sergeant, she supervised detectives in the Criminal Investigations Bureau at Arvada Police Department in Colorado. Dr Charles received her PhD from Saybrook University in the field of Health Psychology in 2005. Having worked in the police community for 27 years, she has recognized the trauma and hardships police officers encounter daily in their profession. Ginger retired from police work in April 2013, teaching psychology at Modesto Junior College in Northern California. Dr Charles is the Executive Director of the Institute For Spirituality & Policing where she continues to research within the police community.

Part IV
Looking to the Future

Chapter 12
Some Futures for the Police: Scenarios and Science

David Weir and Paresh Wankhade

Several chapters in this book, notably those by Neyroud, Rodgers, Meaklin and De Maillard but others also offer perspectives on the future of policing that raise important issues about the nature of police work and the changing societal context. It is not intended to add further complexity to these debates but to essay an overview of these issues which of course do not all point unequivocally in the same direction. In the face of an apparently emerging consensus among insiders and experts, it is worth pointing out that many contentious themes still resonate and are not resolved. Among them are the issues of legitimacy, resourcing and technology.

Some writers (Bradford et al. 2013; Tankebe and Liebling 2013; Hough 2007) point to a current or incipient crisis of legitimacy around questions like whether the public get the police they want or need, and whether these tensions between differing perspectives of what is legitimate as between various publics, the political establishment and the police professionals can be easily resolved. Several writers state as a matter of agreed consensus among experts that the days of street policing are over and public visibility cannot in future be guaranteed, that instant response is always subject to resource limitations and implicit prioritisation of cases (Oliver 2001). This answer makes sense to the expert analyst but there are nonetheless widespread indications that this answer continues to be unacceptable to the public at large (Skogan 2009). It is commonly stated especially at government level that the major threats to security in the UK come from terrorist action, yet in a recent online survey (Greater London Authority 2013, p. 1) about policing priorities faced with a choice between dealing with terrorism or providing safe streets and domestic protection, the responses were 70 % for the latter as a priority.

D. Weir (✉) · P. Wankhade
Edge Hill University, Ormskirk, UK
e-mail: weir53@gmail.com

P. Wankhade
e-mail: Paresh.Wankhade@edgehill.ac.uk

© Springer International Publishing Switzerland 2015
P. Wankhade, D. Weir (eds.), *Police Services*, DOI 10.1007/978-3-319-16568-4_12

Likewise, the emerging establishment view supported by many senior figures in the police service is that "crime is down, crime rates are down and the public should feel reassured". However, it is clear that much of what the public experience as "crime" is not reflected in these statistics (Travis 2014) and that because of "gaming" (which has of course always existed: they were cuffing in Leeds in the 1960s) or explicit suppression many events that are experienced by their victims as highly undesirable are not recorded as crime at all (Patrick 2011; Bevan and Hood 2006).

Neyroud argues that adding back the known quantum of internet and fraud crimes to the acknowledged overt figures would increase these by 50%: these are big numbers and he concludes that the police are failing to cope because of the limitations of geography and political jurisdiction and that this issue challenges legitimacy as well as visible performance (Dry 2014). The grey figure has always been known about, victimless crime has been debated and contended and the widespread existence of white-collar crime has been understood at least since the 1920s, but it is now an undisputed fact that the financial impact of white-collar crime if thoroughly summarised and categorised has vastly overtaken traditional crimes against the person for financial gain. But for one type of crime you lose your liberty for a stretch of years, for another you lose your knighthood and your organisation has to pay something back.

The challenge to the perceived legitimacy of an institution is not always met with at the front door of rational debate but often sneaks in unsuspected through the back door of disillusion or the partly opaque side windows of perception and myth (Maybin 2014). Hard cases make bad law, certainly, but they may stir up strong sentiments. The death of babies due to contaminated feed supplied by a commercial supplier in a specialist unit for the treatment of especially vulnerable cases may make a tiny contribution to an institutional or regional infant mortality rate but its capacity to create an urban myth about societal priorities in a late capitalist urban society may be very powerful. Cases have more impact than rates and if someone in your street has had their private space violated or their body attacked or if one of your hard-working elderly relatives has lost a pension entitlement while fund managers are retiring on six figure salaries to gated communities, the legitimacy issues resonate, perhaps erratically and are capable of amplification in the context of a new politics. In the debate about "fat cats" as well as the de-construction of "Plebgate" alike, for example the Police Federation may no longer continue to be unambiguously respected as the honest broker of professional craft in policing and workers' rights in the face of resource constraints.

As Bishop states in her piece, "The confidence and trust of the public is an absolute priority in policing." The listening skills that Bishop sees as central to the identification of risk depend on the capacity of police and public to meet in the middle for this conversation and the choice of location is driven by the way people live their lives rather than by where the light from the lamppost falls because this is not where the coin was dropped. In encounters with the public procedural justice and efficient outcomes need to be in balance, because research findings show, unsurprisingly but nonetheless significantly that good experiences lead to good perceptions and per contra negative experiences to distrust, cynicism and hostility.

Legitimacy concerns also underlay other issues such as diversity. The Police Foundation and other bodies re-iterate that policing in areas of minority or immigrant populations is inhibited through lack of tacit knowledge about cultural or socio-economic experience but also contributes to lack of perceived legitimacy but some of the suggested solutions like increased recruitment from the international labour market or late onset direct entry of applicants with specialist skills could also exacerbate the legitimacy agenda.

The legitimacy issue does not go away because the experts are satisfied that they can explain how these variances come about. In a period in which the legitimacy of the integrity of the political system called "The United Kingdom" is subject to existential challenge it is highly likely that the legitimacy of other hallowed institutions will continue to be on the public's agenda.

Resourcing issues likewise do not admit of facile solutions. Many writers point out that the glory days of ring fenced budgets for policing are over and will not return. Resourcing lies at the heart of many debates about performance and here again the answers are not simply summarized in increased budgets and clearer outcomes against generic and ultimately unstable pledges about "public confidence". New Public Management and the Performance Culture that produces the Monday Morning review by the "Shudda Brigade" (Marsh et al. 2007) may have faded into the recent history but it is more than the scars that remain.

De Maillard argues that in the French police service, there have been similar impacts on the preference for quantifiable outcomes, increased centralization, increased cynicism, and of course in manipulation of figures and gaming. His recommendation that wider frames of reference than just measurable outcomes, qualitative and softer measures and client and public feedback takes us back into the themes of legitimacy and professionalism. As Rogers points out policing is a "people and information" occupation and to many police people is a true vocation.

The promise of technology enables new systems enabling the police to move from reactive to proactive stances, intelligence-led and systems-driven with the explicit promise that specialist knowledge-bases surmounting geographical limitations and delivered by professionals supported to enhance their capabilities imply that the Skills Agenda needs to be constantly attended to. High profile cases like the Madeleine McCann disappearance and the Ashya King "baby snatching" saga indicate that in terms of some inter-institutional and inter-cultural situations policing in the UK can be portrayed as insular and insensitive.

Language skills, international experience, emotional intelligence and no-blame cultures may be becoming the foundation of experienced operational strategic judgement in the high end glocal labour market and these trends need to be sensed in the police if the service is to move beyond the law and order rhetoric and the founding fundamentals of law, procedure and time served drinking in the tacit knowledge of the canteen culture. Constable and Smith remind us that police cultures are plural and that accommodations to policy changes are likely therefore to be diverse and to some extent unpredictable.

Some historical perspective offers a context. Policing of the kind that we know in the kind of society we thought we were becomes part of the fabric of our society around the same epoch as the printed newspaper in the early-mid Nineteenth century and has arguably been until now rather less disturbed by technology than has the news industry, in which the core delivery model has been dramatically altered by radio, TV, and now by social media. But technology now enables both greater access, integration of delivery systems and personalisation that implicates both news and policing. In most societies there has been an ongoing tussle between individual freedom of access and contestation and the centripetal tendencies of authority, centralisation and hierarchy.

Neyroud further argues that it is police professionals and the police as an evidence-led science who should own the next phase of its future, and many both inside and outside the police service will echo this meme. It is undoubtedly fair to see science as relatively undervalued in this context and as providing the basis for more effective and efficient solutions to operational policing encounters. But it is not clear either that the public en-masse, or as individuals or as represented by the available systems of public control and representation will be ready to cede their extant democratic rights to exert control over their police in this way. The legitimacy issue will not go away.

What many of the contributors to this book have shown is that there exists immense positivity towards the need for a timely re-examination of the fundamentals of policing and the role of the communities and publics they serve. This re-engagement should also encompass the reality of continually-evolving smart technologies that raise the standards of competent performance on both sides of the bargain between publics and police.

What is absolutely certain is that the first movers in "new crimes" like people-trafficking, identity-theft, and communications-interception to name but a few lies with the criminals: both police and public are continually playing catch up. Therefore we may be often too late to catch on because we don't understand the rules of these new games that the criminals are continually making, and perhaps think it beneath our dignity because we "have specialists who know that stuff". A recent McKinsey Report (Divol et al. 2012) on the continuing evolution of information systems in strategic decision concludes that "As artificial intelligence grows in power, the odds of sinking under the weight of even quite valuable insights grow as well. The answer isn't likely to be bureaucratizing information, but rather democratizing it: encouraging and expecting the organization to manage itself without bringing decisions upward." To a great extent discretion in handling roles has always been present in police work, especially perhaps at the level of sergeant where management and street framings of wicked situations admitting no clear protocols are often met and have to be negotiated and implemented using sound judgement based on experience continually updated and necessarily unskilled.

This is already happening in other sectors. In academic life it is now well understood that new technology not only enables existing delivery modes, but fundamentally changes the balance of knowledge-power in the classroom and that the "professor knows best and don't interrupt while he reads his book chapters as a lecture course" model of knowledge transfer leads only to boredom, loss of motivation and untaught students.

Talk of new partnership models of engagement (Maguire and John 2006) must involve downloading tasks into competent and parallel institutional contexts in social services, healthcare, insurance and community organisations for example but also in enabling, enhancing and trusting an increasingly savvy client community to know what they can do for themselves and in moving away from the control and hierarchy-encrusted procedures of the last century and a half. If that creates a new momentum for re-examining the opportunities for prevention of harm, of proactive information-led intervention and for not doing some things that either can't be done with the resource base, don't need to be done because they don't matter or evade the reality of control while delivering big on the rhetoric and the public stance…that may be no bad outcome. The ultimate objective is the good society in which citizens feel safe and criminals feel anxious no matter whose crime figures look good or no matter who takes credit for it. The responsibility for that ultimately lies with both police and the public they serve.

References

Bevan, G., & Hood, C. (2006). What's measured is what matters: targets and gaming in the English public health care system. *Public Administration, 84*(3), 517–38.

Bradford, J., Jackson, J., & Hough, M. (2013). Police futures and legitimacy: redefining good policing. In J. M. Brown (Ed.), *The future of policing*. London: Routledge.

Divol, R., Edelman, D., & Sarrazin, H. (2012). Demystifying social media. *McKinsey Quarterly, 2*, 67–77.

Dry, T. (22nd April 2014). Crime is not falling, it's moved online, says police chief. *The Telegraph*.

Greater London Authority. (2013). *Police and crime plan survey of Londoners*. Summary Report. Greater London Authority: London.

Hough, M. (2007). Policing, New public management and legitimacy in Britain. In T. Tyler (Ed.), *Legitimacy and criminal justice: An international perspective*. New York: The Russell Sage Foundation.

Maguire, M., & John, T. (2006). Intelligence led policing, managerialism and community engagement: Competing priorities and the role of the national intelligence model in the UK. *Policing and Society: An International Journal of Research and Policy, 16*(1), 67–85.

Marsh, C., Weir, D., & Greenwood, W. (2007). *Shudda Brigade: Critical realities of the Sergeant's world of performance management*. Paper presented at the Critical Management Studies Conference, Submission to CMS 5, Manchester Business School, University of Manchester, July 11–13.

Maybin, S. (25th March 2014). Do the public still trust the police? *BBC News Magazine*.

Oliver, W. M. (2001). *Community-oriented policing: A systemic approach to policing* (2nd ed.). New Jersey: Prentice Hall.

Patrick, R. (2011). 'A Nod and a Wink': Do 'Gaming Practices' Provide an Insight into the Organisational Nature of Police Corruption? *Police Journal: Theory, Practice and Principles, 84*(3), 199–221.

Skogan, W. G. (2009). Concern about crime and confidence in the police: Reassurance or accountability? *Police Quarterly, 12*(3), 301–318.

Tankebe, J., & Liebling, A. (2013). *Legitimacy and criminal justice: An international exploration*. Oxford: Oxford University Press.

Travis, A. (24th April 2014). Crime rate in England and Wales falls 15% to its lowest level in 33 years. *The Guardian*.

Prof. David Weir is Visiting Professor at Edgehill University, and has held Chairs at several universities including Glasgow, Bradford, Liverpool Hope, UCS and SKEMA in France. He has worked with several police forces and has published extensively on risk management and undertook a major study with the Police Federation on the work of police sergeants in the UK. He has supervised more than sixty PhD theses on aspects of management and has written several books and many journal articles.

Prof. Paresh Wankhade is the Professor of Leadership and Management at Edge Hill University Business School. He is a founding editor of International Journal of Emergency Services and is recognised as an expert in the field of emergency management. His research and publications focus on analyses of strategic leadership, organisational culture, organisational change and interoperability within the public services with a special focus on emergency services. His publications have contributed to inform debates around interoperability of public services and challenges faced by individual organisations.

Chapter 13
The Future of Policing in the United Kingdom

Timothy Meaklim

Introduction

The art of prophecy is very difficult, especially with respect to the future—Mark Twain

We live in complex times and policing still holds a central role in the maintenance of law and order, however, the public are much more sceptical about the abilities of the police to remedy the problems facing society (Newburn 2012). There is an uncertain future for policing especially with respect to its purpose and organisation. As Crank and Kadleck (2011) state, the organisational concept, practice and function of the police are undergoing transition. Policing does not sit in isolation, but functions in a complex socio-political and operational environment. There is an expansion of policing functions, both due to the escalation of concerns over global issues, but also because policing has now greater involvement with other agencies in dealing with an increasing array of socially related problems which impact on the more traditional criminal problems (Brown 2014). The external factors such as legislation, government policy and the expectations of the public will all influence the future direction of policing. Local, national and international issues will create an ever increasing need for the police to react and alter their strategy to meet these needs. This piece will explore the complexity of policing with special regard to those issues which I consider will influence the future.

T. Meaklim (✉)
University of Ulster, Coleraine, United Kingdom
e-mail: tim.meaklim@yahoo.co.uk

© Springer International Publishing Switzerland 2015
P. Wankhade, D. Weir (eds.), *Police Services*, DOI 10.1007/978-3-319-16568-4_13

Politics and Policing

Government and politics at national, regional and local level all have an impact upon the future shape of policing. National government sets new laws, funding policies and police conditions of service and pay. Individual governments, coalitions and changes in voting patterns all can influence policy on law enforcement and policing, as well as the relationship with the police. Hanley (2014) suggests that the results of the May 2014 elections to the European Parliament were very much as predicted. Frustration with austerity, economic stagnation, diminished opportunities and a yawning sense of disconnect with established parties and politicians, created the environment for a variety of outsider parties to make gains. This discontentment was reflected through the politics of anti-immigration and this tended to benefit right wing, Eurosceptic parties such as United Kingdom Independence Party (UKIP). It is not clear if this is short term movement by voters, however, this discontentment and increased support for right wing politics does increase tension and heightens the possibility of street action and public disorder, as seen in the 2011 London riots.

Reform and Accountability

The coalition government of the Conservatives and the Liberal Democrats set out its plans for police reform in the Home Office consultation document 'Policing in the twenty-first century, reconnecting police and the people' (2010). This proposed Police and Crime Commissioners (PCC), a National Crime Agency (NCA) and the professionalisation of policing. The stated intent was to make the police more accountable, accessible and transparent to the public and therefore make communities safer.

Bradford et al. (2014) suggest that 'the legitimacy of the police is partly about perceptions, and partly about reality. However, improvements in trust and legitimacy have to be earned, and not simply claimed.' The issue of integrity will remain at the forefront of debates especially in light of highly publicised investigations into the behaviours of senior police officers, the police federation and concerns over the recording of crime. The 'Plebgate' scandal, has been one of the most reported of such cases. It concerned an altercation between the Conservative Government Chief Whip MP Andrew Mitchell, and the police at the gate of Downing Street on 19 September 2012. The alleged behaviour of Mr Mitchell resulted in his resignation; however subsequent revelations and investigation by both the Independent Police Complaints Commission (IPCC) and Operation Alice, led by the head of the Metropolitan Police's Directorate of Professional Standards, resulted in a public apology, dismissals and criminal convictions of police officers. In addition lack of openness and transparency by the Police Federation of England and Wales about its affairs and finances led to an Independent Review by the RSA. As a result the Home Secretary Theresa May demanded that the Police Federation reform or be reformed and that the wider police service must address issues of honesty and integrity. Crime statistics published by the Office for National Statistics (ONS) have long been considered central to the understanding of the nature and prevalence of crime in England and Wales. However, the Public Administration Select Committee's inquiry into the UK Statistics Authority (UKSA) decided in January 2014 to strip Police Recorded Crime (PRC) data of its designation as National Statistics (Public Administration Committee 2014). It concluded that the ONS and UKSA had been far too passive about concerns raised and they had missed opportunities to ensure the integrity and quality of PRC data. It also concluded that lax supervision of recorded crime data had reduced the police's effectiveness in their core role of protecting the public and preventing crime. This highlighted a lack of leadership within some sections of the police, and its failure to comply with the values, ethics and integrity expected in Public Life.

Returning to the reform agenda, the Association of Chief Police Officers (ACPO) under pressure from the Home Office, has recognised the need to increase its accountability for what it does and for the public funding it receives. It has been working to create a new governance structure which makes it accountable to those who fund it. In addition the Review of Police Leadership and Training (Neyroud 2010) has resulted in ACPO and the College of Policing developing a framework of national standards and Authorised Professional Practice (APP) which will ensure development is proportionate, targeted at the areas of highest risk and will help to cut crime and increase confidence. The future aspiration is that this will develop the concept of policing as a profession around the world and improve the mobility of expert practitioners, strategies and tactics.

Police and Crime Commissioners (PCC) were introduced in November 2012 in England and Wales (excluding the Metropolitan Police which has separate arrangements). Davies (2014) contends that the policy architecture for the PCC drew inspiration from models of police governance from the USA, which fitted with Conservative views on police reform. Raine and Keasey (2012) suggest that it will take some time for clear, significant and lasting impacts to show themselves. However, the fact that Chief Officers and Crime Commissioners are on limited time due to contracts or re-election means the focus is on short term remedies, rather than long term strategic guidance. The continuation of budgets cuts will mean sustained challenges in setting priorities on the type and quantity of services needed to deliver desired outcomes. This will require the effective and efficient management of existing resources and projects to deliver more with less. As Wheelwright and Clark (1992) state few development projects fully deliver on their promises. They argue that poor decisions and leadership overloads the existing resources and in reality prevents successful completion of the projects. In policing it will be vital to estimate the available resources and prioritise these against the most important projects and pursue only those which will deliver benefit. This will require an on-going reassessment of core and ancillary tasks, along with an assessment of which of these functions requires sworn officers, compared to support officers or civilian staff. Structurally, police services in England and Wales are still primarily organised by geography, with 43 police services. With the creation of Police Scotland the discussion, or many will say the pressure, on regionalisation and force amalgamations will remain.

The final piece of the reform agenda was the introduction of the National Crime Agency (NCA) which became operational in October 2013 with both national and international reach and the mandate and powers to tackle serious and organised crime. Its remit includes border policing, economic crime, organised crime, cyber and cyber-enabled crime and CEOP which tackles sexual exploitation and sexual abuse of children and young people.

Society and Demographics

Broader changes in society and diversity will impact upon future policing arrangements. Coleman (2010) contends that based upon the Office for National Statistics 2008 Principal Projection rates and the ethnic characteristics estimated in his research, the ethnic minority populations will increase from 13 % of the UK population in 2006 to 28 % by 2031 and 44 % by 2056. Twenty five years after the Macpherson Inquiry of 1999, the police service is still being accused of being institutionally racist and not reflecting the communities it serves (Macpherson 1999). While numbers of ethnic minority and female police officers have increased, there is further to go if police services are to reflect and fully understand the communities they serve. The police must consider whether their current strategies adequately encourage those from minority groups, or whether new, creative approaches are required. But, it is not just ethnic changes in society; each generation has particular experiences that mould specific preferences, expectations, beliefs and work style. There are concerns that young people are being alienated from society through high youth unemployment, changes in economics and technology. This needs to be considered alongside the needs of an aging population. The Office for National Statistics estimates that by 2037 the number of people aged 85 and over is projected to be 2.5 times larger than in 2012. Each group requires an appropriate police response supported by Community Safety Partnerships (CSPs) and community policing to improve safety and cohesion.

Police Technology

Technological advances in policing are a vital aspect of modern policing, however often the technology is developed for other purposes and then adapted for police use. This often means that criminals are already ahead in its use. Increasingly technology does support effective and efficient police responses, including:

- Less lethal weapons and tactics have been proven to reduce injuries to both offenders and officers (Smith et al. 2010).

- Global Positioning Systems (GPS) are used for tracking criminals and vehicles and also for resource and fleet management of police vehicles and officers.
- Geographic Information Systems (GIS) help to map and identify crime clusters or threat areas.
- Vehicle mounted, body worn cameras, speed cameras and closed circuit cameras provide methods of detection, verification of incidents and a deterrent to offending.
- Advances in forensic investigation and in particular improvements in the analysis of DNA have become quicker, more effective and cheaper.
- Automatic Number Plate Recognition (ANPR) technology is used to help detect, deter and disrupt criminality including evidence gathering and tackling traveling criminals, organised crime groups and terrorists.
- Mobile applications allow the public to access information advice and services quickly and effectively.

Intelligence and analysis continue to become more sophisticated in policing. For years, businesses have used data analysis to anticipate market conditions or trends and drive sales strategies. Police can use a similar data analysis to help make their work more efficient. Intelligence-led policing has been around for about 15 years. It has increased information sharing, accountability and strategic planning. Beck and McCue (2009) indicate that this can be taken further through a predictive policing model, which can indicate particular times, locations and characteristics predicted to be associated with an increased likelihood for crime. This information can support the prevention, resource allocation, response, training and policy relating to policing. However, the increasing use of technology, surveillance and intelligence brings with it new legal challenges, particularly with regard to the balance between crime control and the private interests of citizens and Human Rights.

Future Threats

Since the London bombings of July 2005, the murder of Drummer Lee Rigby and continued insurgency in parts of the Middle East and North Africa, the threat of terrorism is the most serious danger to face the UK within the last century. Briggs and Birdwell (2009) highlight Muslim communities in the UK have come under intense scrutiny in recent years both as the result of such attacks, but also because of the fear of radicalisation and the emergence of a home-grown threat which raises concerns not just about the future attacks, but it also plays on the deeper anxieties about Britain's growing diversity and apparent loss of a cohesive identity. As Morrow et al. (2013) state the feeling of 'Safety' becomes primarily defined in the negative as the absence or elimination of threat. For policing this creates a balancing act of effective engagement with the Muslim community to support social and political integration against effective counter-terrorism measures to ensure prevention, intelligence gathering and detection of offenders.

McGuire and Dowling (2013) in their review of the UK cyber security strategy noted "a truly robust estimate will probably never be established, but it is clear the costs are high and rising". They state that the costs of cyber crime could reasonably be assessed to equate to at least several billion pounds per year. The increased cyber crime risks extend to many aspects such as:

- financial transactions
- fraud and theft
- identity theft
- sexual offending
- harassment and threatening behaviour
- commercial damage and disorder, and
- targeting the integrity of individual, business and governmental computers and computer networks

Transnational organised crime manifests itself in many forms, including drug smuggling, human trafficking and undermining financial systems through money laundering. As the United Nations Office on Drugs and Crime (UNODC) highlights, organised crime is not stagnant, but adapts as new crimes emerge and as relationships between criminal networks become both more flexible and more sophisticated. It transcends cultural, social, linguistic and geographical borders and must be met with a concerted response from policing and other law enforcement agencies. Too often in the past international co-operation was based upon single incidents and short term tactics. For the future there is a need to develop sustained intelligence and international operational networks.

It is not just crime and disorder that will impact on policing; changes in weather patterns in the UK not only create the immediate problems of flooding or gales, but also impacts on food production, work and transportation. If we also consider pandemics of emerging infectious diseases, health departments generally agree that hospitals and critical care capacity would be overwhelmed even in a mild pandemic or other infectious disease outbreak. But as Brownlie et al. (2006) advocate we need to consider infectious diseases in humans, animals and plants. With global transportation and movement each has the potential to act as a threat to the UK. Although policing will not be the initial lead in these areas, they will need an appreciation of the evolving threat and the factors driving changes in risk and response. In terms of disasters and emergencies, a wide range of groups will need to act through what Koh et al. (2010) refer to as collective socialisation, preparation and efficacy. This requires the highest levels of collaboration, communication and co-ordination before, during and after the crisis.

Developing the Future Policing Response

As discussed earlier, it is not possible to predict the future, but there is the need to explore a vision of the future using a synthesis of information from various techniques. Such an approach encourages planning which as Wilkinson and Kupers (2013) argue can make leaders comfortable with the ambiguity of an open future. They further emphasise that the future is at best a hypothesis rather than a precise data point. Such preparation allows quick adaptation in times of crisis. Leaders can then manage for the unknown and consider appropriate trade-offs. This is about more planning, being more open, transparent and willing to share their resources and experiences (Meaklim 2013). There are a range of methods which can be used to plan and forecast including:

- Evidence- based policing is a research method for making decisions about what works in policing and which practices and strategies accomplish police missions most cost effectively (Sherman 2013).
- Scenario planning is about focusing on the key issues of alternative scenarios for possible events that are crucial to your police service or department. (McGrath and Bates 2013).
- The Delphi forecasting method explores issues to get expert consensus (RAND Corporation 2014).
- SWOT analysis is used to summarise the Strengths, Weaknesses, Opportunities and Threats facing policing (Pahl and Richter 2007).
- PESTEL stands for—Political, Economic, Sociological, Technological, Legal, and Environmental. It is an audit of an organisation's environmental influences with the purpose of using this information to guide strategic decision-making (McGrath and Bates 2013)

Increased planning and research allows greater integration between academics, researchers and practitioners. This approach encourages theory and practice to be interwoven and supports testing, innovation and flexibility.

Final Thoughts

Relying on old paradigms for the future will make it impossible to deliver an effective, efficient and meaningful service to the community. Complexity in policing has increased due to a combination of globalisation, technology, demography and the world financial crisis. As Newburn (2012) points out policing has changed, as has the society being policed and the pace of change is increasing. One way or another, we must consider what it is we want policing in general and the police service in particular to achieve to meet these changes. Whilst working to maintain the sources of stability and continuity policing needs the ability to shape and build development capabilities, both at individual and organisational level. Good leadership is fundamental to high performance in uncertainty and in the future the need will be greater than ever. Meaklim and Sims (2011) highlight the need of leaders to be able to think on the go, make tough choices, recognise patterns among different types of problems, search for facts to prove or disprove hypothesis, draw on one's own knowledge and the knowledge of others and work collaboratively to imagine and shape the future.

References

Beck, C., & McCue, C. (2009). Predictive policing: What can we learn from Wal-Mart and Amazon about fighting crime in a recession? *The Police Chief,* LXXVI, 11. (November 2009).

Bradford, B., Jackson, J., & Hough, M. (2014). Police futures and legitimacy: Redefining good policing. In J. M. Brown (Ed.), *The future of policing* (pp. 79–100). Oxon: Routledge.

Briggs, R., & Birdwell, J. (2009). *Radicalisation among Muslims in the UK*. MICROCON Policy Working Paper 7. Brighton: MICROCON

Brown. J. M. (2014). *Future of policing*. Oxon: Routledge.

Brownlie, J., Peckham, C., Waage, J., Woolhouse, M., Lyall, C., Meagher, L., Tait, J., Baylis, M., & Nicoll, A. (2006). *Foresight. infectious diseases: Preparing for the future—Future threats.* London: Office of Science and Innovation.

Coleman, D. (2010). Projections of the ethnic minority populations of the United Kingdom 2006–2056. *Population and Development Review, 36*(3), 441–486.

Crank, J., & Kadleck, C. (2011). *Policing: toward an unknown future*. Oxon: Routledge.

Davies, M. (2014). The path to police and crime commissioners. *Safer Communities, 13*(1), 3–12.

Hanley, S. (2014). When anger masks apathy. UCL European Institute. http://www.ucl.ac.uk/european-institute/highlights/2013-14/ep2014-cee. Accessed 14 June 2014.

Home Office. (2010). *Policing in the 21st century, reconnecting police and the people: consultation*. London: The Stationery Office.

Koh, H., Cadigan, R., Kawachi, I., Subramanian, S., & Kim, D. (2010). *Social capital and health* (p. 274). New York: Springer Science.

Macpherson, W. (1999). *The Stephen Lawrence inquiry report*. London: HMSO.

McGrath, J., & Bates, B. (2013). *The little book of big management theories, and how to use them.* England: Pearson.

McGuire, M., & Dowling, S. (2013). *Cyber crime: A review of the evidence. Home Office Research Report 75*. London: Home Office.

Meaklim, T. (2013). Considering game theory to improve leadership in partnership working within the UK public services. *International Journal of Leadership in Public Services, 9*(1/2), 22–31.

Meaklim, T., & Sims, J. (2011). Leading powerful partnerships—A new model of public sector leadership development. *The International Journal of Leadership in Public Services, 7*(1), 21–31.

Morrow, D., McAlister, B., Campbell, J., & Wilson, D. (2013). Mediated Dialogues and systematic change in Northern Ireland. Policing Our Divided Society 1996–2003. University of Ulster Institutional Repository. http://eprints.ulster.ac.uk/27681/. Accessed 8 June 2014.

Newburn, T. (2012). *Handbook of policing*. 2nd ed. Cullompton: Willan.

Neyroud, P. (2010). *Review of police leadership and training*. London: Home Office.

Pahl, N., & Richter, A. (2007). *Swot analysis Idea, methodology and a practical approach*. Germany: Druck and Bindung.

Public Administration Committee. (2014). Caught red-handed: Why we can't count on Police Recorded Crime statistics. http://www.publications.parliament.uk/pa/cm201314/cmselect/cmpubadm/760/76003.htm. Accessed 24 June 2014.

Raine, J., & Keasey, P. (2012). From police authorities to police and crime commissioners: Might policing become more publicly accountable? *International Journal of Emergency Services, 1*(2), 122–134.

Rand Corporation. (2014). The delphi model. http://www.rand.org/topics/delphi-method.html?page=1. Accessed 11 June 2014.

Sherman, L. W. (2013). *The rise of evidence-based policing: targeting, testing, and tracking. Center for Evidence-Based Crime Policy (CEBCP)*. Chicago: The University of Chicago.

Smith, M., Kaminski, R., Alpert, G., Fridell, L., MacDonald, J., & Kubu, B. (2010). *A multi-method evaluation of police use of force outcomes: Final report to the National Institute of Justice*. USA: U.S. Department of Justice.

Wheelwright, S., & Clark, K. (1992). Creating project plans to focus product development. *Harvard Business Review, 70*(2), 70–82. (March—April 1992).

Wilkinson, A., & Kupers, R. (2013). Living in the futures. *Harvard Business Review, 91*(5), 119–127. (May 2013).

Dr Timothy Meaklim is a Management and Learning Consultant. He has a wide range of experience in leadership, research and education within policing both within the UK and internationally. He has a particular interest in ensuring that learning is transferred to the workplace and makes an impact on organisational effectiveness. Timothy is an Associate Lecturer in Strategic Leadership in the School of Criminology, Politics and Social Studies, University of Ulster.

Chapter 14
Future Perspectives in Policing: A Crisis or a Perfect Storm: The Trouble with Public Policing?

Peter Neyroud

In the early years of the twenty-first century, public policing in the developed world has been going through a very rough patch. Whether it be riots in London, riots in Ferguson, Missouri resulting from a police shooting, a series of scandals in the UK both historic and current (May 2014) or just the deep impact of financial austerity following recession, policing and police leaders have tended to be making the news for the wrong reasons. For one UK commentator the institutional crisis was so deep-rooted that nothing short of abolition would cure the problem. Professor Tim Hope (2014) stated his case based on the harms caused by public policing, such as the discriminatory impacts of policies such as stop and search, the culture of policing, which he suggested is insular and self-serving and on the lack of police effectiveness in their main mission of crime control.

Hope could also have pointed out that, alongside his arguments, there was a "perfect storm" affecting public policing across the developed world (Neyroud and Weisburd 2014). Firstly, most countries have experienced a level of financial austerity not seen since the oil crisis of the 1970's. Policing budgets have been cut in the UK, Europe and the USA. Long-term projections of the impact of demographic changes suggest that, although debt and falling tax revenues caused the immediate cuts, the future looks very challenging (Gascon and Fogelsong 2010): a future that public policing must face with an institutional structure with embedded inefficiencies (Van Reenen 1999). Despite technological changes, police budgets the world over show that around 80 % of expenditure remains committed to the cost of the workforce, a figure that has not changed in 30 years. Proportionate to other public sector agencies, policing has become more expensive just at the time when it needs to reduce costs (Gascon and Fogelsong 2010).

P. Neyroud (✉)
Jerry Centre for Experimental Criminology, Institute of Criminology,
Cambridge University, Cambridge, UK
e-mail: pwn22@cam.ac.uk

© Springer International Publishing Switzerland 2015
P. Wankhade, D. Weir (eds.), *Police Services,* DOI 10.1007/978-3-319-16568-4_14

Given the costs of policing, it is, therefore, particularly problematic that the second dimension of the "storm" is the challenge of demonstrating the effectiveness of the police as crime falls and its patterns change. In an international debate about the reasons for the crime drop, few analyses of the causes have accorded police a central role. The most convincing explanations advanced have suggested that situational crime prevention—engine immobilisers, better home security and surveillance technologies - has been more effective (Van Dijk 2014). Furthermore, as police numbers have fallen, there has, as yet, been no consequent uplift in recorded crime figures.

One reason why official figures are not rising is that those figures increasingly fail to reflect the changes in crime patterns. The Office for National Statistics (ONS) has estimated that more than 3 million fraud and Internet based crimes go unrecognized by both official figures and the Crime Survey of England and Wales (ONS 2014). Added to the official tally, these crimes would provide an increase of around 50 % in the UK. The police are simply failing to cope, because they remain locked into a geographic model of policing with physical boundaries and nationally defined legal remits. The police are also struggling to cope with crimes such as people trafficking, child sexual exploitation and domestic violence, which cross the boundaries of countries, agencies or public and private space. The solutions are too often posed as structural reorganization of the existing organisation rather than a more fundamental realignment (Curtis 2014). Ultimately, this existential crisis of policing is challenging the legitimacy of the police as an institution. Far from enjoying a "Cold War" dividend from the crime drop, the public police have faced renewed scrutiny about their mission, purpose and contribution (Neyroud and Weisburd 2014).

In the past the police would, no doubt, have fallen back on experience and traditional law and order rhetoric. With increasingly tough choices between funding health, education, defence and other public services, such an approach is unlikely to win many arguments. Police leaders need a much more radical strategy to sustain their services and prevent what George Kelling has called the "retreat to the core" (Police Executive Research Forum PERF 2012), which would push public policing more and more to an unattractive future as an emergency service of last resort for struggling communities. Indeed, Brogden and Ellison (2013) have argued that the piecemeal responses of police leaders to austerity have already started the slide in such a dystopic direction.

There is an alternative approach. Even those commentators who have minimized the contribution of the police and focused on the impact of the wider safety and security web in encouraging changes in behaviour (by victims and offenders) through regulation, prevention and rehabilitation, have found room for better policing as a driver of past and continued reductions (Waller 2014). In doing so, Waller (2014) and other key authors have argued that a reliance on experience and traditional tactics are not sufficient. Instead, Laycock and Tilley (2002) have proposed a renewed attention to "professional" problem-solving", Waller (2014) advocated a "smarter crime control" focusing on "problem places and problem people" (p. 52) and Sherman (2013) a "Triple T" strategy—targeting, testing and tracking—using the best evidence available. The common strand to each of these is a conception of the future of policing as a new profession, using knowledge to support delivery and innovation and research to test, learn and develop effective practices (Neyroud and Sherman 2013).

Reforming the police service along these lines is not an easy proposition. Police education remains stubbornly rooted in a model largely defined in the nineteenth century in which law and procedure combined with the passing on of experience are given preference over evidence based practice (Neyroud 2011; Weisburd and Neyroud 2011). Furthermore, the old police professional model, based around O.W. Wilson's scientific management (Wilson 1950), was condemned for placing too much reliance on the three R's—random patrol, rapid response and reactive investigation –, which were all shown to be relatively ineffective by the research in the 1970's and 1980's (Skogan and Frydl 2004). A new professionalism would have to pay more attention to public engagement, evidence and strategies focused on enhancing legitimacy (Travis and Stone 2011).

For police leaders confronting the challenges of the "perfect storm", Neyroud and Weisburd (2014) and Neyroud and Sherman (2013) have argued that the essential task is for police to own, deploy and develop the science of policing. Ownership in this context includes the police embracing science (in its widest sense of knowledge) as the key building of practice and investing in partnership with scientists (the academic community) to build and enhance that knowledge. For this to happen, police officers and police leaders will need to value science as a key determinant of their choice of tactics and strategy and a vital part of the qualification framework for any applicant to or practitioner in policing.

An example of how such an approach changes the police is presented by the debate about the use and deployment of Body Worn Video (BWV). The idea that police should extend surveillance of their operations from the interview room into the wider operational environment is not a new one. The Royal Commission on Criminal Justice (1993) oversaw a test of operational tape recording as early as 1992. New technologies mean that more 20 years on, many of the physical constraints have been overcome. Too often such technologies have then been introduced without proper testing and evaluation and with more attention paid to the operation of the technology than to the social and societal impacts of their use. Instead, a serving Chief supported by an academic partner led a randomised controlled trial into BWV (Ariel and Farrar 2014). The RCT involved all the officers in Rialto Police Department being randomly assigned to wear or not wear BWV. The outcomes demonstrated a significant reduction in assaults on officers and complaints of misconduct by officers where the equipment was being worn. The study has encouraged a wider debate and further studies to replicate and broaden the profession's understanding (PERF 2014).

The growing body of research and systematic reviews of research in policing now provide the profession of policing with an agenda, which is very different from the 3 R's model of the 1950's (Rapid response, reactive investigation and random patrol). The police can be effective if they focus their efforts on high crime places or hot-spots, on highly recidivist and harmful offenders and on protecting the most vulnerable victims (Sherman 2013). By paying attention to the impact of each approach or the combination of approaches on their perceived legitimacy, the police should be able to avoid the backfire effects of over-intensive deterrence based approaches (The Crime Report 2014). By extending the science to prevention and deterrence challenges such as cybercrime and organised crime, police could start to reframe their role at the heart of the state's duty to protect the citizen from preventable harms. Retreating to the core, on the other hand, could threaten the institutional extinction provocatively laid out by Hope (2014).

References

Ariel, B., & Farrar, J. (2013). *The Effects of Body Worn Video on Police Citizen Encounters: An RCT*. Presentation to the 2013 Conference on Evidence-based policing: www.crim.ac.uk/events/ebp/2013. Accessed 1 April 2015.

Brogden, M., & Ellison, G. (2013). *Policing in the age of austerity*. London: Routledge.

Curtis, I. (2014). *Speech to the Superintendents Association of England and Wales Annual Conference 2014*. http://www.policesupers.com/presidents-speech-structures-blame-culture-welfare/. Accessed 1 April 2015.

Gascon, G., & Fogelsong, T. (2010). *Making the Police more affordable*. https://www.ncjrs.gov/pdffiles1/nij/231096.pdf. Accessed 1 April 2015.

Hope, T. (2014). *I would give up 0... the police service*. http://www.crimeandjustice.org.uk/resources/i-would-give-police-service. Accessed 1 April 2015.

Laycock, G., & Tilley, N. (2002). *Working out what to do: Evidence-based crime reduction. Crime Reduction Series Research Paper 11*. London: Home Office.

May, T. (2014). *Speech to the Police Federation Conference 2014*. https://www.gov.uk/government/speeches/home-secretarys-police-federation-2014-speech on 15/09/2014. Accessed 1 April 2015.

Neyroud, P. W. (2011). *Review of police leadership and training.* London: Home Office.

Neyroud, P. W., & Sherman, L. W. (2013). Dialogue and dialectic: Police legitimacy and the new professionalism. In J. Tankebe & A. Liebling (Eds.), *Legitimacy and criminal justice: An international exploration*. Oxford: Oxford University Press.

Neyroud, P. W., & Weisburd, D. (2014). Transforming the police through science: Some new thoughts on the controversy and challenge of translation. *Translational Criminology, Spring*, 16–18.

Office for National Statistics. (2014). *Crime in England and Wales, year ending March 2014*. http://www.ons.gov.uk/ons/rel/crime-stats/crime-statistics/period-ending-march-2014/stb-crime-stats.html. Accessed 1 April 2015.

PERF (2012). *Is the economic downturn fundamentally changing how we police?* Washington, DC: Police Executive Research Forum.

PERF (2014). *PERF and COPS Office to release report on Body Worn Video*. Subject to Subject Debate July/August 2014. http://www.policeforum.org/assets/docs/Subject_to_Debate/Debate2014/debate_2014_julaug.pdf. Accessed 1 April 2015.

Royal Commission on Criminal Justice. (1993). *Cm 2263*. London: HMSO.

Sherman, L. W. (2013). The rise of evidenced-based policing: Targeting, testing and tracking. In M. Tonry (Ed.), *Crime and justice in America 1975–2025*. Chicago: University of Chicago Press.

Skogan, W., & Frydl, L. (2004). *Fairness and effectiveness in policing*. Washington, DC: National Academies Press.

The Crime Report. (2014). *The Crisis of Confidence in Police Community Relations*. http://www.thecrimereport.org/news/inside-criminal-justice/2014-09-the-crisis-of-confidence-in-police-community-relation. Accessed 1 April 2015.

Travis, J., & Stone, R. (2011). *Towards a new professionalism in Policing*. http://www.hks.harvard.edu/var/ezp_site/storage/fckeditor/file/pdfs/centers-programs/programs/criminal-justice/ExecSessionPolicing/NPIP-TowardsaNewProfessionalisminPolicing-03-11.pdf. Accessed 1 April 2015.

Van Dijk, J. (2014). Presentation to Crime Seminar for University of Sheffield, 27th February 2014.

Van Reenen, P. (1999). The "unpayable" police. *Policing: An International Journal of Police Strategies & Management, 22*(2), 133–152.

Waller, I. (2014). *Smarter crime control: A guide to a safer future for citizens, communities and politicians*. Lanham: Rownham and Littlefield.

Weisburd, D. W., & Neyroud, P. W. (2011). *Police science: Towards a new paradigm*. Washington, DC: Department of Justice, National Institute of Justice.

Wilson, O. W. (1950). *Police administration*. New York: McGraw-Hill.

Prof. Peter Neyroud CBE, QPM served for 30 years as a police officer in Hampshire, West Mercia, Thames Valley (as Chief Constable) and the National Policing Improvement Agency (as CEO). In 2010, he carried out the "Review of Police Leadership and Training" which led to the establishment of the new "National College of Policing", in 2012. Since 2010, he has been a Resident Scholar at the Jerry Lee Centre for Experimental Criminology at the Institute of Criminology, Cambridge University. As an affiliated lecture and research manager, he has been doing a PhD, managing a major research programme at Cambridge University and teaching senior police leaders and advising governments across the world. He is a Visiting Professor at Chester University and Edgehill Universities, a Visiting Fellow at Nuffield College, Oxford, Teesside University and Buckinghamshire New University and a Research Associate at the Oxford Centre for Criminology. He is a Trustee Board Member of the Internet Watch Foundation. He was awarded the Queens Police Medal in 2004 and a CBE in the Queen's Birthday Honours List in 2011.

Chapter 15
International Perspectives in Policing: Challenges for 2020

Colin Rogers

Introduction

Anticipating the future can be a challenge. Forecasting future events clearly involves the risk of error and one should always be aware of the possibilities of such mistakes being made. Despite this, when considering the subject of the future of policing one thing is certain. Policing does not exist in a vacuum (Dolling 2003). It is impacted upon daily and in the long term, by changes in the social, political, economic, technological, environmental and legal structures, in whatever country it is practised. It therefore follows that the future structure and activities of policing will be shaped by the future changes within these categories and this is an appropriate place to start with our considerations.

In particular, policing is a 'people and information' occupation. Therefore police leaders and managers in all countries need to clearly understand how population can trend. Further, there is a need to understand how information is gathered, exchanged and utilised, and the consequences of these activities. Globalisation, and the global economy, is now characterised by the almost instantaneous flow and exchange of information, capital and cultural communication (Castells 2010). The increasing nature and scope of crime and substantial increases in immigration tend to demonstrate that, what happens in one country can have an impact in others.

C. Rogers (✉)
International Centre for Policing and Security, University of South Wales, South Wales, UK
e-mail: colin.rogers@southwales.ac.uk

© Springer International Publishing Switzerland 2015
P. Wankhade, D. Weir (eds.), *Police Services*, DOI 10.1007/978-3-319-16568-4_15

International Trends

According to the National Intelligence Council in the USA, (National Intelligence Council 2008), the world's population will reach 8 billion by 2025, up from 6 billion in 2000. However, this increase will not occur evenly across all countries. Developed countries will see a decline in population whilst those of developing countries will increase, particularly in Sub-Saharan Africa and South Asia, which will have extremely youthful populations. Developed countries will witness an aging population rise, coupled with declining fertility rates, leading to less individuals of working age to support the population as a whole. Workers have to come from somewhere; as a consequence we may witness a large expansion in immigration and shifts in population from one country to another. In terms of social changes then, such a population shift—which increases both migration and immigration—will bring with it the attendant risk of internal and external change within different societies. For example, the above population shift could bring about an expansion of the 'middle classes' across different countries, which could lead to an expansion of the consumerist society already witnessed in most Western countries to the global stage (Spybey 1996). This in turn could lead to a higher demand from communities for more service oriented, citizen/consumer style policing (Clarke et al. 2009), rather than a law enforcement model of policing as people come to understand their rights as consumers of private and public services.

Urbanisation is set to grow to about 60% in all countries (National Intelligence Council 2008) which will require not only a concentration of policing services within those areas, but may also elicit a decline in social cohesiveness, which is required to support and promote 'self policing'. This has been part of a continuing responsibilisation strategy for most democratic governments for some time within communities (Garland 2001).

Rapid political changes, coupled with wider social movements, are likely to exist which might produce serious governance difficulties. There may be wider democratisation which will lead to greater calls for transparency and accountability in policing agencies across the globe, coupled with greater franchise. This could occur despite the possibility of increased nationalism. Clearly the political landscape will be far more complicated in the future than hitherto.

In terms of economic changes, the recent economic recession witnessed in developed countries across the world may last longer than anticipated. What we may witness is that Asia will surpass North America and Europe in global economic power.

Perhaps the biggest area of change for international policing by the year 2020 will be seen in the greater use and expansion of more and more sophisticated technology on a global stage. Not only will it influence organisational behaviour and crime trends, but it will also impact upon individual and personal lifestyles. Developments in technology will further enhance the potential for greater and swifter communication between groups of people who are able to organise themselves for dealing with such activities as political protest, whilst the potential for global crime, such as terrorism, will increase exponentially. Schafer et al. (2005, 2012) suggest the following major challenges for the police in terms of the current trends in technology:

- New types of crime will come into being
- Traditional crime will become enhanced by new technologies
- There will develop a technology gap with the police falling further behind the private sector in understanding and acquiring new technologies.

Whilst new technology provides challenges for police, it can also provide benefits. For example, improvements in data analysis tools, biometrics and less lethal technologies provide enhancements for police activities.

One cannot ignore the fact that increased problems for policing agencies may occur as a result of environmental and climate change. The recent large scale bush fires in Australia, extensive floods in UK and elsewhere in the world, and severe snow storms in the USA, may indicate that natural disasters could increase in scale and intensity. Increased opportunities for global travel may increase the possibility of a worldwide pandemic. These potential environmental problems will in turn require different and varied responses at a national and international level, and a greater need and demand for closer cooperation between police agencies with more and wider services across the world.

Due to the continuing mantra of 'more for less' or even 'less for less' in the delivery of policing services within developed countries, we may witness increased amounts of legislature in an attempt to compensate for and deal with citizens in the absence of government sponsored police, and the possible rise of greater policing activities by private sector security agencies. Clearly, more crime prevention activities will need to be in place, with the possibility of greater use of surveillance, and situational crime prevention techniques, rather than costly social interventions. The challenge for all policing agencies will be that of providing and stimulating a need for greater social cohesion/community involvement (Rogers 2012; Wedlock 2006) in the delivery of policing services due to the 'thinning out' of previously well-funded police organisations. This enhanced cooperation and partnership approach with communities will be vital in order to maintain the very legitimacy that allows for policing in democracies.

Old Structures Challenged

Like most modern organisations, police agencies in Western countries trace their origins to the country's industrial revolution and, consequently, their structures are similar, with workers being supervised by an overseer within a hierarchical structure that separates front line officers from strategic policy makers (Hebdon and Kirkpatrick 2006). The paramilitary model of policing does not adapt well to external demands for change or accountability, and there is still a tendency to adhere to historical ideas regarding management practices. Therefore, policing agencies in developed countries are in need of a revolution in their organisation, leadership and management models in order to deal with the future issues that they will have to face. Paradoxically, countries wishing to develop their policing services, such as those in Africa and South America as well as other parts of the world, still seek to develop their policing agencies in line with traditional Western countries. For example, the concept of community policing, whether rhetoric or reality, (Greene and Mastrofski 1988) is an appealing one for countries seeking to legitimise their policing process, especially when tourism or leisure economics are seen as a way of developing growth and security. However, the very idea of the Western or democratic style and structure of policing is itself in need of enormous change, and therefore developing countries and other international police agencies need to appreciate and understand the potential impact of future trends upon traditional police structures.

Challenges for Police Leadership

For developing and developed countries alike, leadership skills for police will need to be adjusted to meet the potential challenges that are likely to occur. Technology and financial links, coupled with increased travel technology, means that threats and risks are constructed on a global landscape as well as locally, regionally and nationally. An understanding of such, and an appreciation of how structures are connected at the global level, will be an important skill for police leaders in whatever country they are situated. Further, an ability to manage change at short notice, coupled with complex abilities such as an understanding of research methods, mastering and understanding technological changes and trends will be required. Factors that impact upon national and international law and an ability to integrate strategy, culture and political concerns within the organisation will also be required skills. In particular, as a framework surrounding all of these changes and ideas, police leaders of today need to understand that they were trained in a substantially non changing, bureaucratic structured organisation which has resulted in an organisational culture with sometimes displays fixed attitudes, and that this structure will need to be changed in order to meet the challenges of the future.

References

Batts, A. W., Smoot, S. M., & Scrivner, E. (2012). Police leadership challenges in a changing world. http://ncjrs.gov/pdffiles1/nij/238338.pdf. Accessed 13 March 2014.
Castells, M. (2010). *The rise of the network society* (2nd ed.). Chichester: Wiley-Blackwell.
Clarke, J., Newman, J., Smith, N., Vidler, E., & Westmarland, L. (2009). *Creating citizen-consumers: Changing publics and changing public services*. London: Sage.
Dolling, D. (2003). *Community policing: Comparative aspects of community policing orientated police work*. Reiden: Felix-Varlag.
Garland, D. (2001). *The culture of control: Crime and social order in contemporary society*. Oxford: Oxford University Press.

Greene, J. R., & Mastrofski, S. D. (1988). *Community policing: Rhetoric or reality*. New York: Praeger Publishers.

Hebdon, R., & Kirkpatrick, I. (2006). *Changes in the organisation of public services and their effects on employment relations*. In S. Ackroyd (Ed.), *The oxford handbook of work and organisation*. Oxford: Oxford University Press.

National Intelligence Council. (2008). Global trends 2030. http://www.dni.gov/files/documents/GlobalTrends_2030.pdf. Accessed 12 March 2014.

Rogers, C. (2012). *Crime reduction partnerships*. Oxford: Oxford University Press.

Schafer, J. A. (2005). Policing 2020, exploring the future of crime, communities and policing. http://fwg.cos.ucf.edu/publications/Policing2020.pdf. Accessed 12 March 2014.

Schafer, J. A., Buerger, M. E., Myers, R. W., Jensen, C. J., & Levin, B. H. (2012). *The future of policing, A practical guide for police managers and leaders*. Boca Raton: CRC.

Spybey, T. (1996). *Globalisation and world society*. Cambridge: Polity.

Wedlock, E. (2006). Crime and community cohesion, Home Office report 19/06. http://webarchive.nationalarchives.gov.uk/20120919132719/ http://www.communities.gov.uk/documents/communities/pdf/452513.pdf. Accessed 13 March 2014.

Prof. Colin Rogers is Head of Research at the International Centre for Policing and Security at the University of South Wales, UK, and a Visiting Professor at Charles Sturt University, NSW, Australia. A former UK police officer with 30 years' service he has researched nationally and internationally for different police agencies on areas such as community policing, organisational change and police education and has published extensively on diverse matters concerning policing. He is the current editor of The Police Journal: Theory, Practice and Principles.

Chapter 16
International Perspectives in Policing: Challenges for 2020

Jacques de Maillard

Introduction

At all levels of police administration, the use of performance indicators is common currency, both internally (the monitoring and management of personnel) and externally (exchange of information with partners, police communication). It is undeniable however that numerical data has assumed a wider scope due to the extension of new management techniques within these organizations, as well as due to the budgetary rationalization affecting all European countries over the recent years. The introduction of new public management tools, the technological transformations related to the diffusion of new software and the political pressures for increased accountability have combined their effects to spread these new performance tools in police organisations, albeit with a certain number of variety among countries (J. de Maillard and Savage 2012).

The present piece proposes to review the effects of the measure of performance through indicators on police services through the specific example of the French national police. If quantified indicators have existed for long, they have been massively used since the 2000's with the introduction of a managerial approach based on a "culture of results" or "performance". The article first analyses the effects associated to the measurement of performance and then proposes some solutions in the management of police services.

J. de Maillard (✉)
CESDIP and Institut Universitaire de France, University of Versailles-Saint-Quentin,
Versailles, France
e-mail: jdemaillard@gmail.com

© Springer International Publishing Switzerland 2015
P. Wankhade, D. Weir (eds.), *Police Services,* DOI 10.1007/978-3-319-16568-4_16

Performance Indicators and Police Activity

Large amount of literature has empirically documented the perverse and unintended effects of the introduction of performance indicators in England and Wales (especially Hough 2007; Loveday 2006; Patrick 2011) as well as in the US (Eterno and Silverman 2012). Our empirical findings for the French national police are very much in line with this strand of research (de Maillard and Mouhanna 2015). More particularly, four effects appear:

Firstly, due to the use of performance indicators, the substance of police activity has focused on quantifiable activity, i.e. essentially on crime, at the expense of solving daily problems, a kind of activity that is more difficult to quantify. Police action has been centred on what was more easily measurable, hence on crime and clearance statistics. Practices of targeting have been developed for the benefit of measurable goals or easy investigations that enabled results to be improved.

Secondly, the development of performance indicators has often resulted in the increased centralization of the police organization, inducing a top-down logic and greater control from above rather than promoting collective learning and decentralization. Despite official rhetoric linking performance and accountability, the use of performance indicators in the 2000's has in fact increased centralization in three ways: the operationalization of objectives, the establishment of rewards and sanctions, and the monitoring of daily activities.

Thirdly, this single focus on crime figures also developed some cynicism within the police by leading agents to concentrate on the measurable often leading to stress. This logic also had the effect of limiting partnership practices (Matelly and Mouhanna 2007) because they were harder to measure.

Finally, the pressure of numbers has generated an accentuated recourse to various forms of numerical juggling (Bevan and Hood 2006) which call into question the integrity of the police. The usual by-products have been various forms of under–recording of criminality (with various stratagems to dissuade complainants or manipulation to remove masses of complaints from official statistics), practices that have been denounced by administrative inspections (IGA-IGPN-IGGN-IG Insee 2013).

An Eightfold Path to a More Reflexive Use of Performance Indicators

Despite their perverse effects, there are serious grounds to consider that the use of performance indicators won't diminish in the future. The technological advances will translate into new software more comprehensive in terms of data available and more users-friendly. The political pressure and its consequences in terms of managerial accountability should continue. Hence, thinking about challenges for 2020 involves taking into account this trend and reflect on how to adapt it to improve the quality of the police organizations. We outline here an approach in 9 different components. These include, broad definition of performance, qualitative criteria, performance processes, sense making, professionalism, long-term approach, localism, and problem-solving. Each of them is explained next in some details.

Firstly, the police should adopt a **wider rather than narrower definition of performance**. If by performance, we understand "good policing"; it is necessary to adopt a more global approach of how performance should be measured. Senior police officials must be particularly careful to think of the police in a broader way and take into account the potential perverse effects of performance management. An approach of the police activity in terms of legitimacy is a central requirement (Bradford et al. 2013). Therefore performance indicators should not be limited to crime and should not be only internal to the police. Let us recall that in most continental countries for instance, contrary to England and Wales, there is no measure of users' satisfaction (let us think that is even a measure of confidence in London). Scoreboards should be balanced to go beyond the sole police activity related to crime.

Secondly, the police managers should pay attention to the "**qualitative" dimension**. The notion of "quality" is difficult to define (and it may explain why police organisations remain cautious about using it), but it refers to a part of activity that is not easily reducible to quantified indicators. Let us take an example: a police agent may have a large number of arrests, it doesn't tell us anything about the quality of these arrests (the percentage of arrests resulting in a charge on the repressive, quality of the interaction with the person arrested on the human side, etc.). Quality means to have a finest evaluation of the performance of the various police segments. In consequence, supervision in the police organisation can't be reduced to the monitoring of quantified indicators: it implies to know how work is achieved concretely.

This leads us to the third correlate: "**results**" (defined for instance in terms of declining crime rate) as such are not a sufficient indicator of performance. An agent (or an organisation) may reach targets because he/she/it is lucky. Therefore, importance must be given to **processes** as well as results. What are the processes (in terms of analysis, strategy design, evaluation, etc.) at work to deal with a specific problem? Police officers should be responsible for their outputs rather than outcomes, for the quality of their processes rather than their rough results.

Fourth, statistical data don't give as such any **meaning to police activity**. The role of managers at every level of the hierarchy is to give sense to the activity of their subordinates. To be leaders, in the most general meaning of the term, they must be able to give a sense (in terms of police activity) to their subordinates. Data facilitate analysis and support strategy, but numbers can't as such constitute a strategy.

Fifth, the previous points imply that the police should be based on the **professionalism** of its agents. The risk of management by numbers has been to increase centralisation and take out responsibilities from agents. Standards of professionalism (with specific skills, competences and personal qualities) should be defined, in which discretion could be exercised. Standards of professionalism should be given priority over organisational constraints.

Sixth, due to the transformation of data systems, the "numbers" (i.e. quantitative indicators on the various aspects of police activity such as crime trends, clearance rate, resources available, etc.) are more and more available on a short-term basis. Police officers, at every level of the hierarchy may check their "results" on a daily level, with all the negative consequences associated to this practice. Police analysts and managers must analyse crime trends, define **mid-term objectives**, fix problems in a sustainable manner and don't give in to temptation of short-term results.

Seventh, the risk with the use of performance indicators is that when data is manipulated, inaccurate and gives false evidence on reality. The more data are decontextualized, the more they may be wrongly interpreted. Data should be interpreted in a specific context. Centralised management may neglect this necessary contextualisation of data. **Local context** is essential in solving police problems.

Eighth, **solving problems** implies often multi-organisational practices. The use of performance indicators must avoid a closing of the police organisation on itself. Police administrators must reflect on the limits of their own indicators, think of joint indicators with their partners. In other words, to better serve and protect, the police will have to be particularly cautious, reflexive and not heed the siren song of easy-to-measure performance indicators.

In conclusion, the lessons are particularly true for the French national police where the focus on the "culture of results" or of "performance" has led to a impoverished definition of what police performance should be. But these lessons have a broader reach (see for England, among others, Hough 2007 or, for New York, Eterno and Silverman 2012). Performance indicators are a means of police performance, not an end. They must provide information, help to elaborate strategies and to evaluate actions undertaken. The words of caution of Herman Goldstein—the "means over ends" syndrome—have kept their accuracy: "All bureaucracies risk becoming so preoccupied with running their organizations and getting so involved in their methods of operating that they lose sight of the primary purposes for which they were created. The police seem unusually susceptible to the same phenomenon" (1979, p. 236). The easiness to manipulate performance indicators risks oversimplifying police activity. Problem solving, long-term approach, localisation, professionalism are essential conditions of contemporary "good policing".

References

Bevan, G. & Hood, C. (2006). What's measured is what matters: Targets and gaming in the English public health care system. *Public Administration, 84*(3), 517–538.

Bradford, J., Jackson, J. & Hough, M. (2013). Police futures and legitimacy: Redefining good policing. In J. M. Brown (Ed.), *The future of policing*. London: Routledge.

De Maillard, J., & Savage, S. (2012). Comparing performance: The development of police performance management in France and Britain. *Policing & Society, 22*(4), 363–383.

De Maillard, J., & Mouhanna, C. (2015). Governing the police by numbers. In J. Ross & T. Delpeuch (Eds.), *The democratic governance of intelligence: New models of participation and expertise in policing*. Stanford: Stanford University Press.

Eterno, J., & Silverman, E. (2012). *The crime numbers game. Management by manipulation*. New York: CRC.

Goldstein, H. (1979). Improving policing: A problem-oriented approach. *Crime and Delinquency, 25*(2), 236–238.

Hough, M. (2007). Policing, new public management and legitimacy in Britain. In T. Tyler (Ed.), *Legitimacy and criminal justice: An international perspective.* New York: The Russell Sage Foundation.

IGA-IGPN-IGGN-IG Insee. (2013) L'enregistrement des plaintes par les forces de sécurité intérieure, report n 13051-13027-1. http://www.interieur.gouv.fr/Publications/Rapports-de-l-IGA/Securite/ Rapport-sur-l-enregistrement-des-plaintes-par-les-forces-de-securite-interieure. Accessed 1 April 2015.

Loveday, B. (2006). Policing performance: The impact of performance measures and targets on police forces in England and Wales. *International Journal of Police Science & Management, 8*(4), 282–293.

Matelly, J.-H., & Mouhanna, C. (2007). *Police. Des chiffres et des doutes.* Paris: Michalon.

Patrick, R. (2011). A 'nod and a wink': Do 'gaming practices' provide an insight into the organizational nature of police corruption? *The Police Journal, 84,* 199–221.

Jacques de Maillard is Professor of Political Science at the University of Versailles-Saint-Quentin, deputy-director of the Cesdip (a research centre affiliated to the CNRS, the University of Versailles and the ministry of Justice) and at the Institut Universitaire de France. His interests lie in the issues of governance of security, plural policing, police reforms and the comparative study of policing in European countries. He has recently published "Comparing performance: the development of police performance management in France and Britain" (with S. Savage), Policing & Society, 22 (4), 2012, pp. 363–383 and Projecting national preferences: police co-operation, organizations and polities" (with A. Smith), Journal of European Public Policy, 19 (2), 2012, pp. 257–274.

Erratum

Chapter 1

Introduction: Understanding the Management of Police Services

Paresh Wankhade and David Weir

P. Wankhade, D. Weir (eds.), *Police Services,* DOI 10.1007/978-3-319-16568-4_1

The Publisher regrets that chapter 1 had several errors in the printed version and now the correct version of chapter 1 has been typeset again and attached after erratum page.

The online version of the original chapter can be found under
http://dx.doi.org/10.1007/10.1007/978-3-319-16568-4_1

Paresh Wankhade
Edge Hill University, Ormskirk, UK
e-mail: Paresh.Wankhade@edgehill.ac.uk

David Weir
Edge Hill University, Ormskirk, UK
e-mail: weir53@gmail.com

Introduction and Background

This book is the first of a three volume series on the management of the three blue light emergency services (Police, Ambulance and the Fire & Rescue Services) being published by Springer, USA. This volume aims to provide a broader management understanding of the police services which would be of equal interest to a wide audience including students, academics, practitioners, professionals including the leadership & management practitioners in police forces without compromising the rigour and scholarship of the content. We have invited experts in their particular fields to address the chosen themes, both in the theory and practice of the functioning of the police services in the UK and abroad. The key thinking in this volume is to provide a broad understanding of the major management issues relevant to police services in the UK along with an international perspective. Admittedly it is a difficult endeavour to cover all the possible management themes in a single volume such as this but we are confident that the chosen topics will provide an expert view and a rounded understanding and insights into the management of police services.

More attention is being paid now to the management research on police services given the policy and practice implications of the challenges and changing context of policing. Several factors have contributed toward the need for a better understanding of the role and contribution of the police services in the wider criminological settings. The pressures on police budgets and the resulting implications for service delivery have been well rehearsed. The deteriorating global security climate and the growing numbers of cyber-crime cases coupled with lower public confidence and low staff morale is likely to add more pressures on the use of the police services. The Mid Staffordshire Hospital Inquiry (Francis 2013) and the Keogh Review (NHS England 2013) both highlighted a cultural transformation of the hospital and emergency/urgent care services in England. This calls for a similar understanding of the police services thus making this project particularly timely. The chosen themes in this volume will help to outline the social, cultural, and political context in which the police services is to be understood. This volume covers issues of theory, policy and practice and raises questions, some of which are intrinsically controversial. Each of the chapters seeks to engage with the current debates about the direction of travel. The contributors also examine the latest development in their chosen field of enquiry. This volume thus aims to set out the management understanding of the police services as a significant sub-discipline of emergency management and also provide a basis of learning and teaching in this field.

P. Wankhade (✉) · D. Weir
Edge Hill University, Ormskirk, UK
e-mail: Paresh.Wankhade@edgehill.ac.uk

D. Weir
e-mail: weir53@gmail.com

Changing Context of Policing

In the UK, we are currently witnessing two contradictory trends: that of decline in the policing and crime statistics in the UK amidst escalation of global violence, and the growing threats to world security climate. The international peace is threatened by a range of events, sometimes not connected but each posing a significant policing challenge and having implication for an appropriate police response. For instance, the turmoil from the continuing civil war in Syria, the latest round of escalation of violence in the Arab-Israel conflict including the deteriorating situation in Iraq and the rise of a new militant group are a few cases to note. Another totally unconnected danger is from the pandemic threat of the new deadly *Ebola Virus* from West Africa, posing a significant challenge to policing with global ramifications.

In the UK, the latest Crime Survey in England and Wales (CSEW) for the year ending March 2014 revealed that there were an estimated 7.3 million incidents of crime against households and resident adults (aged 16 and over) for the year ending March 2014 (see Fig. 1.1). This represents a 14% decrease compared with the previous year's survey and is the lowest estimate since the CSEW began in 1981 (Office for National Statistics ONS 2014). However, this is in contrast with the police recorded crime figures which show no overall change from the previous year, with 3.7 million offences recorded in the year ending March 2014. Prior to this police recorded crime figures have shown year on year reductions since 2002/2003 (ONS 2014).

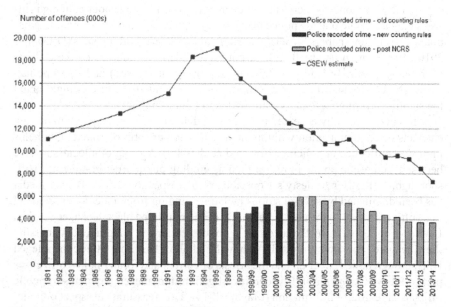

Fig. 1.1 Police recorded crime, 1981 to 2013/14. (Source: Office for National Statistics-Crime in England and Wales, Year Ending March 2014)

There is no consensus among experts about the reasons for fall in the crime figures and a range of factors including the decline in binge drinking, rising alcohol prices and the state of the economy have been reported (Travis 2014). Jon Boutcher, the national policing spokesman on surveillance was reported (Dry 2014) to argue that drop in crime figures was misleading since lot of criminal behaviour has moved online, where much of it goes either unreported or undetected and warned of being complacent to the dangers of cyber-crime. Furthermore, the CSEW (previously British Crime Survey) in use since 1982 has undergone changes from being a research tool to be seen as a system of performance management (Hough et al. 2007). Significant methodological limitations of using surveys as research tools in measuring the performance of public services have been reported (Cantor and Lynch 2000). Recently, Feilzer (2009) examined whether the data collected through the BCS (now CSEW) can be considered as valid and reliable indicators of local police performance. Her analysis showed that perceptual measures included in the BCS and used as performance measures are 'under-conceptualised, invalid, context dependent, strongly related to social-demographics and are unreliable'.

Meaningful performance reporting by police forces and in wider public services has been under considerable scrutiny (Shane 2010; Wankhade and Barton 2012; Loveday 2008; De Bruijn 2002; Wankhade 2011; Andrews and Wankhade 2014) with the MORI 2007 survey (IPOS MORI 2008) reporting how a large proportion of public do not believe crime is falling and more than 60 % of the public have not heard of the Police Inspection Agency (Her Majesty's Inspectorate of Constabulary). The Casey Report (2008) describes that less than 1 % of respondents relied on published statistics as their primary source of information to find out whether the crime in their region was increasing or decreasing. Information about policing is increasingly available outside police agencies through different sources including national TV and newspapers, official websites, and social networking sites (O'Connor 2010). Research on factors that drive public confidence conducted by the College of Policing (formerly National Policing Improvement Agency) and Metropolitan Police (NPIA/Home Office Final Report 2010; Neyroud 2010) further highlighted the significance of good quality information put out to public.

It has been generally accepted that opening dialogue with public and improving channels of communication with public acts as another form of contact and helps improve confidence in policing (Bradford et al. 2009). A string of allegations have been levelled at the police in recent months eroding public trust in policing (Hillsborough, 2012; Her Majesty's Constabulary of Inspection 2011). British media has been dominated by several stories including ranging from undercover Scotland Yard officers trying to influence the family of the murdered black teenager Stephen Lawrence in London, to the arrest of a police officer for lying about witnessing the "Plebgate" row involving MP Andrew Mitchell in Downing Street; the alleged Hillsborough police cover up and the arrests of current and former police officers as part of the Met's Operation Elveden investigation into alleged payments to public officials in return for information (Maybin 2014). The 'reassurance' aspect of policing offers another perspective in improving public confidence (Skogan 2009).

Police services are also witnessing a new challenge on the institution of the Police Federation of England and Wales which is a staff association for all police constables, sergeants and inspectors. An Independent Review led by Sir David Normington (2014) has provided a series of recommendations (pp. 65–68) to improve trust and accountability, foster openness and transparency and improving financial priority with a detailed timetable to re-write the terms and reference of the federation's constitution. Furthermore, acting on a whistle-blower's case from the Metropolitan Police Service, the House of Commons Public Administration Select Committee (PASC) published a damning report about the massaging of the Police Recorded Crime statistics (PASC 2014). The report recommended to the UK Statistics Agency (UKSA) acting in response to the evidence exposed by PASC's inquiry, to strip Police Recorded Crime statistics of the quality designation 'National Statistics' (PASC 2014, p. 52).

Historically, concerns over police accountability and the control of wide ranging police discretion impacting on individual's civil liberties are as old as policing itself (Feilzer 2009; Gains and Cains 1981; van Maanen 1973). A 'tripartite' structure of police accountability which distributed responsibilities between the Home Office, the local police authorities and the chief constable of the force was in vogue till recently. In November 2012, 41 Police and Crime Commissioners (PCCs) were publicly elected across England and Wales, something billed as the most significant constitutional reform in the last five decades. The PCCs became responsible for a combined police force area budget of £ 8 billion to hold Chief Constables and the force to account; effectively making the police answerable to the communities they serve (Association of Chief Police Officers ACPO 2014). The real impact of the elected PCCs on accountability relationships is still being debated (Keasey and Raine 2012; Sampson 2012; Joyce 2011) with Lister (2013) arguing that the new 'quadripartite' governance framework for police institutional accountability may generate pressures on PCCs to interfere in what Chief Constables do.

Important lessons are to be learned by the police services from the Frances report (NHS England 2013) into the patient deaths at the Mid Staffordshire NHS Foundation Trust which re-emphasised the need for organisations to create and maintain the right culture (Foster 2003) to deliver high-quality care that is responsive to users' needs and preferences. Loftus (2010) argued that the underlying world view of officers displays remarkable continuity with older patterns, and police culture endures because the basic pressures associated with the police role have not been removed questioning the increasingly accepted view that orthodox conceptions of police culture no longer make any sense. Many of these changes will require a different style of policing, one which "fosters the trust and confidence of local communities and meets their concerns and expectations" (Karn 2013, p. 5). Understanding police culture(s) nevertheless offers important insights into the nature of the organisation and how it deals with issues of legitimacy, accountability and future direction of travel (Waddington 1999; Barton 2003; O'Neil et al. 2007; Cockcroft 2013).

Against the changing landscape of policing, the role and function of the police is also changing. The police mission has become broader and more complex, embracing functions more commonly associated with other agencies (Karn 2013). Yet the public (and political) expectation from police services still centres on crime protection. This volume provides a timely discussion of some of the key management issues being confronted by the police services.

Aims and Plan of this Book

This volume provides a mature understanding of an important public service. Thus, one of the aims of this volume is to invite a new generation of management scholars to explore the study of the police services. This volume will also appeal to a range of students (both undergraduate and postgraduate) studying organisational theory as well as social sciences, sociology, economics and politics, community engagement, emergency planning and disaster management. The book offers critical insights into the theory and practise of strategic and operational management of police services and the related professional and policy aspects. For a large number of staff working in the emergency care settings, the growing calls for professionalisation of the service (through closer links with Higher Education Institutes HEIs) and the recognition to reflect on their own personal development, this volume seeks to provide an authoritative source on the management of the police services addressing the knowledge gaps. This volume will equally appeal to a growing audience of independent practitioners and consultants, both in the UK and working around the world.

One of the other aims of this volume is to bring together, top-quality scholarship using experts- academics, practitioners and professionals in the field, to each of the chosen topics. Admittedly this was an ambitious task and we have been really fortunate to have an assembly of authors who are well regarded for the expertise in their fields. They range from senior academics, chief constables, serving and ex-police officers & police staff, and independent practitioners. To bring them all together is a key highlight of this volume and to this end this is a book by the people who lead and manage the police services and their opinions is important in informing the policy and guiding the practice. The contributors have written from different perspectives of critical academics to chief executives and policy experts and there is much to be gained from reading chapters in 'conjunction with each other, contrasting different perspectives and approaches' (Newburn 2003, p. 7). We are immensely grateful to them for their untiring work that has gone to produce this volume and feel confident that it will do justice to the complexities of the chosen themes. All the chapters have been completed in 2014 and hence draw upon the latest evidence and research base available on the chosen topic. The chapters are based in the practical experiences of the authors and are written in a way that is accessible and suitable for a range of audiences.

In dealing with these issues, the volume is divided into four parts. Part I provides the context and background to this volume. Chap. 1 examines the context of policing and states the aims of this volume. In Chap. 2, John G.D. Grieve explores the historical perspectives in policing. His chapter looks back to the founding fathers of policing in the 18th and 19th Centuries and considers whether their thinking has any application in the governance reforms of the early twenty-first Century. He provides a practitioner's reflective view of where policing came from and what is the significance for governance, leadership and management now of those earliest days? He argues in his piece that Robert Peel deserves much of the credit for the practical development of the emerging framework, even if not the precise labelling of them as Peel's *Nine Principles of Policing* that he has sometimes been given. But he should be given the credit as an artificer building on what had been begun earlier rather than as a completely original thinker as Douglas Hurd's work advises us (Hurd 2007). Reith's articulation remains helpful as an ideal. These Principles, he concludes, have relevance and find resonance even today.

Part II of this volume deals with the 'doing' of the police services in preventing crime and providing order in the society. Six key themes are examined. In Chap. 3, police leadership is examined by Andrew Fisher and John Phillips. They argue that the police services are facing a crisis of public confidence amidst a range of current challenges. The service is being faced, not only, with political and fiscal challenges, but also cultural & structural problems, and societal issues have threatened the principles of policing by consent and legitimacy. They contend that the crisis can be seen to be the result of failed leadership and policing strategies over decades, and the danger is that there will be more of the same. Case for a new model of policing that recognises the value of engaging communities to re-build confidence and assist in the single mission of reducing crime, based on 'trust, norms and networks' is made in their piece. This chapter examines the challenges and explores what needs to be done to make this happen.

In Chap. 4, Julian Constable and Jonathan Smith examine the contentious theme of police occupational culture. The study of police occupational culture has revealed a wealth of hitherto unknown and unseen aspects of the working life of police officers. In the social science literature this culture is often linked to many of the problems that have been evident in the police organisations of England and Wales. In this way, the authors argue, initial training environment is often considered a place where otherwise 'good' new recruits are inducted into a sub-culture that is pernicious to themselves, the service and those they police. The case study of initial training described in their piece, indicates a complex picture where examples of practice and behaviour that is both progressive and problematic are found. Some specific recommendations are made with regard to changes that might be considered for future iterations of initial police training by the force in question and the service as a whole.

In Chap. 5, the issue of community engagement is investigated by Susan Ritchie. She argues that adopting a deficit model of public service delivery where services 'fix' communities rather than build on the strengths they have, is just not working. She provides a personal practitioner perspective of the future of democracy in the UK with a particular focus in the way public services understand the communities they serve. Going beyond public confidence and satisfaction ratings more democratic initiatives such as Citizens' Charters, pledges and local area agreements offer greater opportunity to reconnect the state with the individual and to re-think the feminist phrase of 'the personal is political' so that it can be applied to all public services. She concludes that by developing new skills to listen differently to the communities they serve, police services can act as the 'enablers' of active citizenship to reduce demand and improve social capital.

In Chap. 6, Rowland Moore explores the issue of equality and diversity in police forces in a short piece. He argues that being immersed in a culture dominated by people who might be different by gender, sexuality, race or disability, presents significant additional personal challenges. Some are obvious from the outset and are by definition easier to deal with whereas others are more insidious involving practices seemingly ingrained in organisational culture. He contends that in the final analysis, policing appears to be heavily populated by values underpinned in conservatism—a political philosophy or attitude emphasizing respect for traditional institutions, distrust of government activism and opposition to sudden change in the established order. In Chap. 7, Andrea Bishop examines the 'frontline' view of the management of risk in policing. For her, strong leadership and operational credibility are crucial components for senior managers to readily possess and to successfully deliver against in policing. She argues that confidence and trust of the public is an absolute priority and is at the heart of British policing. Members of the public will always turn to the police in times of need and it is in these difficult times that we must ensure that we get it right. She concludes that a proactive approach to listening coupled with strong leadership can help to make sensible decision about addressing risks and managing them.

In Chap. 8, Jon Murphy explores the essence of policing from his perspective of a Chief Constable in the North West of England. He argues that the police service has always been excellent at training its people; investing huge amounts of money and resources on how to do 'stuff', about the law, codes of practice, about process and the tactical delivery. But whilst they train well, they are not so good at teaching people to think about policing, about its mission and its legitimacy. From him, there is nothing revolutionary or clever about the basic philosophy of policing, but quite the opposite-"I don't believe in fixing what is isn't broken and I don't believe in change for change sake." Notwithstanding various challenges, not least of shrinking budgets, he concludes that police forces maintain and build on their reputation by keeping the public safe, and by being openly accountable for their actions.

Part III of the volume explores current debates in policing through three key themes. The issue of police accountability is examined by John W Raine in Chap. 9. The election across England and Wales in November 2012 of 41 Police and Crime Commissioners (PCCs)—one for each police force area outside London marked the launch of an intriguingly novel approach to police governance at the local level. The new arrangements have replaced the tradition of committee-style model, originally of council-led 'police committees', and subsequently (from 1964) of separate 'police authorities' (comprising a mix of nominated councillors and other local appointees). The new PCCs are directly-elected individual office-holders whose role it is to provide the strategic leadership and democratic governance for police and crime-related activity, including the key role of holding the chief constable and the local police force to account on behalf of the public. Drawing from empirical analysis of interviews with a sample of PCCs, the various accountability relationships are evaluated. It is concluded that each of the PCCs was also driven by desire to acquire good personal understanding of public expectations about policing and crime reduction and to ensure that such understandings could be reflected in their own prioritisations of policing resources and in their approach to the role more generally.

Our next author Barry Loveday deals with the subject of police modernisation in Chap. 10. His key argument is that the future police management in an age of austerity should be ready to experiment with innovative developments that provide a level of service expected of it by the public. The modernisation debate cannot be about police establishment any longer but should concentrate on both police deployment and more effective resource allocation. He argues that if the evidence suggests that further reductions in police establishment, when balanced by increases in non-sworn civilian staff undertaking more operational roles could increase police effectiveness, then this should be addressed. It is further contended that in an environment that now increasingly recognises the significance and impact of anti-social behaviour on both individuals and communities, there is a clear case for further evaluation of alternatives to a police response to it. The chapter suggests some possible avenues which could provide the basis for both an effective collaboration between police and local authorities while also providing a more effective response to community demands and victim's needs.

The subject matter of 'personal resilience and policing is next examined in Chap. 11 by our experts Jonathan Smith and Ginger Charles. Police services around the world face many kinds of challenges which often impact directly, and not always positively, on the people who work within these organisation. These are often manifested through increasing levels of stress, burnout and PTSD (Post traumatic stress disorder). In this chapter the authors have explored how resilience may be useful in assisting people to not only cope with these challenges but thrive and prosper in this environment of uncertainty and rapid and constant challenge and change. The chapter develops further, the idea of holistic resilience, and explores the component parts to this, using a holistic framework called the Global Fitness Framework. It investigates some of the benefits to developing greater resilience at individual, organisational and societal level and concludes with an exploration of how the different elements to resilience might be developed by police organisations.

Part IV of this volume presents perspectives on the future of the police services, both in the UK and internationally. Rather than long chapters, these contributions are intended to be shorter pieces to capture greater variety and expertise surrounding the future of policing. The first contribution by David Weir and Paresh Wankhade provides a counter-view on the arguments put forth by some of our contributors on the future of policing and is discussed in Chap. 12. They also comment about the nature of police work and the changing societal context for policing. The piece contends that some of these debates do not all point necessarily in the same direction and many contentious themes still resonate and are not resolved notwithstanding an emerging consensus among police officers and experts. They raise the issues of legitimacy, resourcing and technology and argue that the ultimate objective for everyone should be a society in which citizens feel safe and criminals feel anxious.

They conclude that the responsibility for that ultimately lies with both police and the public they serve.

In Chap. 13, Timothy Meaklim argues that in complex times policing still holds a central role in the maintenance of law and order. There is an uncertain future for policing especially as the organisational concept; practice and function of the police are undergoing transition. His piece explores the current complex socio-political, technical and operational environment of policing, before considering possible key topics that will impact upon the future of policing including terrorism, cyber-crime, organised crime and threats created by climate change or infectious diseases. Finally it considers how leaders and the police organisation can forecast, plan, and manage the future policing response to meet the changing environment, whilst remaining flexible and able to work through uncertainty.

Our next expert opinion in Chap. 14 is provided by Peter Neyroud who draws attention to a deep crisis in public policing which has been precipitated by the combination of fiscal austerity, falling crimes and changing crime patterns. He argues that the crisis is affecting the legitimacy of the institution and requires a new approach from police leaders. To him, the new approach centres around the police taking ownership of the science of policing and building new professional practice based around evidence and supported by a reformed police education. For this to happen, he contends, that the police officers and police leaders will need to value science as a key determinant of their choice of tactics and strategy and a vital part of the qualification framework for any applicant to or practitioner in policing. For police leaders confronting the challenges of the "perfect storm", it is essential task for police to own, deploy and develop the science of policing.

In Chaps. 15–16, we present two contributions addressing international perspectives for police services. In Chap. 15, Colin Rogers argues that policing is not a stand-alone activity, but is affected by many different global changes and other social factors. Consequently police leaders now and in the future will need to be aware of potential global activities in order to provide an adequate response to changing circumstances. Further, police organisations will need to be flexible and adapt to these changes in order to remain effective. This chapter considers the potential changes and their impact that will provide future challenges for police leaders. In Chap. 16, Jacques de Maillard, exploring the French National Police, argues that at all levels of police management, the use of dashboards and performance indicators is usual, both internally to manage personal and vis-à-vis external partners. His text aims to question the effects of the uses of these indicators by taking the example of the French National Police. After having briefly described the modes of operation of police organizations affected by the deployment of these indicators, he analyses the impact on police work and interactions within the police organisation as well externally. The piece especially focuses on the rationalisation process at work, the perverse effects associated to these new policy instruments and the internal controversies associated to them.

Limitations of the Current Project

As editors there were a few difficult decisions we had to take; the biggest one was to decide what to include in the volume of this and what was to be excluded. We are also conscious about the possible disagreements about the final contents of the volume and what else could or should have been covered. Furthermore, even the scope of some of the chapters could have been more detailed and capable of being examined in a greater detail. The chosen themes do not aim to cover the whole gamut of issues which could be applied to the management of police services. Nonetheless they provide a fair representation of topics that concern us in our scholarly research and teaching. We firmly believe that they represent opportunities for both teaching and practice to reflect on these issues. We also seriously deliberated upon the choice of the authors and their backgrounds. In the end we were convinced that a choice reflecting a balance between academic experts and senior practitioners would bring greater criticality and reflection to the understanding of the chosen themes. Rather than having rigid guidelines over chapter style and structures, we saw greater relevance in a 'light touch', free flowing style of each of the chapters in presenting the contrasting perspectives from academics and practitioners. We are of the opinion that this approach worked better in a work like this though it will be for our readers to judge whether we were correct in our methodology. Similarly we could have paid more attention to the developments in policing outside England though there remains a strong comparative element from Europe.

Future Research Agenda

Police services play a crucial role in maintaining order in the society and in preventing crime. But the context in which they currently operate within the criminal justice system is increasingly becoming fragmented, complex and politically contested. The challenges of funding, training, online-crimes and cultural transformation are now felt globally. The need to learn and adapt from suitable models of police service delivery across the globe have never been greater. We sincerely hope that this volume will trigger greater interest in the understanding of one of the most important of public services. We aim to further work on a comparative element outside the UK and invite interested colleagues and partners to join the quest of the management understanding of a service which is so important to the society.

References

Andrews, R., & Wankhade, P. (2014). Regional variations in emergency service performance: Does social capital matter? *Regional Studies*. doi:10.1080/00343404.2014.891009.
Association of Police and Crime Commissioners (2014). Role of the PCC. Available at http://apccs.police.uk/role-of-the-pcc/ (accessed 7 September 2014).

Barton, H. (2003). Understanding occupational (sub) culture- a precursor for reform: The case of the police service in England and Wales. *International Journal of Public Sector Management, 16*(5), pp. 346–358.

Bradford, B., Jackson, J., & Stanko, E. (2009). Contact and confidence: Revisiting the impact of public encounters with the police. *Policing & Society, 19*(1). pp. 20–46.

Cantor, D, & Lynch, J. P. (2000). Self-report surveys as measures of crime and criminal victimisation. *Criminal Justice,* 4, pp. 85–138.

Casey, L. (2008). *Engaging communities in fighting crime,* crime and communities review. London: Cabinet Office.

Cockcroft, T. (2013) *Police cultures: Themes and concepts.* Oxon: Routledge.

De Bruijn, H. (2002). *Managing performance in the public sector.* London: Routledge.

Dry, T. (2014) Crime is not falling, it's moved online, says police chief. *The Telegraph,* 22nd April 2014.

Feilzer, M. Y. (2009) Not fit for purpose! The (Ab-) use of the British crime survey as a performance measure for individual police forces. *Policing, 3*(2), pp. 200–211.

Foster, J. (2003). Police cultures. In Newburn, T (eds)., Handbook of Policing. Willan: Cullompton, Chapter 9, pp. 196–227.

Francis, R. (2013). *Mid staffordshire NHS Foundation trust public inquiry. Final Report.* London: The Stationery Office.

Gaines, L. K., & Cain, T. J. (1981). Controlling the police organization: Contingency management, program planning, implementation and evaluation. *Police Studies: An International Review of Police Development, 16,* pp. 16–26.

Her Majesty's Constabulary of Inspection. (2011). *Without fear or favour: A review of police relationships.* London: HMIC.

Hillsborough Independent Panel. (2012). *Hillsborough the report of the Hillsborough independent panel.* London: HC 581, The Stationery Office.

Hough, M., Maxfield, M., Morris, B., & Simmons, J. (2007). The British crime survey over 25 Years: Progress, problems, and prospects. In M. Hough & M. Maxfield (Eds.), *Surveying crime in the 21st century.* Cullompton: Willan.

Hurd, D. (2007). Robert Peel. Weidenfeld and Nicolson:London.

IPOS MORI. (2008). *Closing the gaps crime and public perceptions. Ipsos MORI.* London: Social Research Institute.

Joyce, P. (2011). Police reform: From police authorities to police and crime commissioners. *Safer Communities, 10*(4), pp. 5–13.

Karn, J. (2013). *Policing and crime reduction: The evidence and its implications for practice.* London: Police Effectiveness in a Changing World Project, Police Foundation.

Keasey, P., & Raine, J. W. (2012). From police authorities to police and crime commissioners. *International Journal of Emergency Services, 1*(2), pp. 122–134.

Lister, S. (2013). The new politics of the police: Police and crime commissioners and the 'operational independence' of the police. *Policing, 7*(3), pp. 239–24.

Loftus, B. (2010). Police occupational culture: Classic themes altered times. *Policing and Society, 20*(1), pp. 1–20.

Loveday, B. (2008). Performance management and the decline of leadership within public services in the United Kingdom. *Policing: A Journal of Policy and Practice, 2*(1), pp. 120–130.

Maybin, S. (2014). Do the public still trust the police? *BBC News Magazine,* 25th March 2014.

Newburn, T. (2003). *Handbook of policing.* Cullompton: Willan.

Neyroud, P. (2010). Protecting the frontline: The recessionary dilemma. *Policing, 4*(1), pp. 1–6.

Normington, D. (2014). *Police federation independent review: Final report, The trusted voice for frontline officers, The Royal Society of Arts.* London: RSA.

NHS England (2013). Transforming Urgent and Emergency Care in England: Urgent and Emergency Care Review, Phase 1 Report, NHS England: Leeds.

NPIA/Home Office Final Report. (2010). *The national workforce modernisation programme.* London: The Stationery Office.

O'Connor, D. (2010). Performance from the outside. *Policing, 4*(2), pp. 152–156.

Office for National Statistics. (2014). *Crime in England and Wales, Year Ending March 2014, Statistical Bulletin*. London: ONS.

O'Neill, M. E., Marks, M., & Singh, A. (2007). Police occupational culture: New debates and directions. *Sociology of Crime Law and Deviance*, Vol. 8. Emerald.

Public Administration Select Committee. (2014). *Caught red-handed: Why we can't count on police recorded crime statistics. Thirteenth report of session 2013–14. HC 760*. London: The Stationery Office.

Sampson, F. (2012) Hail to the chief? How far does the introduction of elected police commissioners Herald a US-Style politicization of policing for the UK? *Policing, 6*(1), pp. 4–15.

Shane, J. M. (2010). Performance management in police agencies: A conceptual framework. *Policing: An International Journal of Police Strategies & Management, 30*(1), pp. 6–29.

Skogan, W. G. (2009) Concern about crime and confidence in the police: Reassurance or accountability? *Police Quarterly, 12*(3), pp. 301–318.

Travis, A. (2014). Crime rate in England and Wales falls 15% to its lowest level in 33 years. *The Guardian*, 24th April 2014.

Van Maanen, J. (1973). *Observations on the making of policemen*. Cambridge: Massachusetts Institute of Technology.

Waddington, P. A. J. (1999). Police (canteen) sub-culture: An appreciation. *British Journal of Criminology, 39*(2), pp. 287–309.

Wankhade, P. (2011). Performance measurement and the UK emergency ambulance service: Unintended Consequences of the ambulance response time targets. *International Journal of Public Sector Management, 24*(5), pp. 384–402.

Wankhade, P. & Barton, H. (2012). Conceptualising a police performance framework in an era of financial constraint. *Policing Today, 18*(3) pp. 44–46.

Prof. Paresh Wankhade is the Professor of Leadership and Management at Edge Hill University Business School. A former civil servant specialising in indirect taxation, he is a founder Editor of International Journal of Emergency Services (an Emerald group Publication) and is recognised as an expert in the field of emergency management. His research and publications focus on analyses of strategic leadership, organisational culture, organisational change and interoperability within the public services with a special focus on emergency services. His publications have contributed to inform debates around interoperability of public services and challenges faced by individual organisations.

Prof. David Weir is Visiting Professor at Edgehill University, and has held Chairs at several Universities including Glasgow, Bradford, Liverpool Hope, UCS and SKEMA in France. He has worked with several police forces and has published extensively on risk management and undertook a major study with the Police Federation on the work of police sergeants in the UK. He has supervised more than sixty PhD theses on aspects of management and has written several books and many journal articles.

Index

© Springer International Publishing Switzerland 2015
P. Wankhade, D. Weir (eds.), *Police Services,* DOI 10.1007/978-3-319-16568-4

Printed in the United States
By Bookmasters

Printed in the United States
By Bookmasters